MARIJUANA AS MEDICINE?

The Science Beyond the Controversy

ALISON MACK
JANET JOY

for the Institute of Medicine

NATIONAL ACADEMY PRESS
Washington, D.C.

NATIONAL ACADEMY PRESS • 2101 Constitution Avenue, N.W. • Washington, D.C. 20418

NOTICE: The project that is the subject of this report was approved by the Governing Board of the National Research Council, whose members are drawn from the councils of the National Academy of Sciences, the National Academy of Engineering, and the Institute of Medicine. The Principal Investigators responsible for the original report were chosen for their special competences and with regard for appropriate balance.

This book was supported by a grant to the Institute of Medicine by the Robert Wood Johnson Foundation. Any opinions, findings, conclusions, or recommendations expressed in this publication are those of the author(s), and the Robert Wood Johnson Foundation does not take responsibility for any statements or views expressed.

PRINCIPAL INVESTIGATORS AND ADVISORY PANEL FOR IOM REPORT: The following people served as principal investigators and advisors to the 1999 IOM report, *Marijuana and Medicine: Assessing the Science Base*, on which this book is based:

JOHN A. BENSON, JR., *co-Principal Investigator*, Oregon Health Sciences University School of Medicine, Portland; STANLEY J. WATSON, JR., *co-Principal Investigator*, University of Michigan, Ann Arbor; STEVEN R. CHILDERS, Wake Forest University, Winston-Salem, North Carolina; J. RICHARD CROUT, Crout Consulting, Bethesda, Maryland; THOMAS J. CROWLEY, University of Colorado, Denver; JUDITH FEINBERG, University of Cincinnati Medical Center, Cincinnati, Ohio; HOWARD L. FIELDS, University of California in San Francisco; DOROTHY HATSUKAMI, University of Minnesota, Minneapolis; ERIC B. LARSON, University of Washington Medical Center, Seattle; BILLY R. MARTIN, Virginia Commonwealth University, Richmond; TIMOTHY VOLLMER, Yale School of Medicine, New Haven, Connecticut

Library of Congress Cataloging-in-Publication Data

Mack, Alison.
    Marijuana as Medicine? : the science beyond the controversy / Alison Mack, Janet Joy.
        p. cm.
    Includes bibliographical references and index.
    ISBN 0-309-06531-3
    1. Marijuana—Therapeutic use. I. Joy, Janet E. (Janet Elizabeth), 1953-. II. Title.
RM666.C266 M325 2000
615'.32345—dc21

                                        00-046058

Additional copies of this report are available from National Academy Press, 2101 Constitution Avenue, N.W., Lockbox 285, Washington, D.C. 20055; (800) 624-6242 or (202) 334-3313 (in the Washington metropolitan area); Internet, http://www.nap.edu

Printed in the United States of America

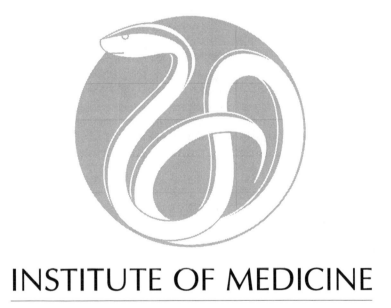

INSTITUTE OF MEDICINE

Shaping the Future for Health

THE NATIONAL ACADEMIES

National Academy of Sciences
National Academy of Engineering
Institute of Medicine
National Research Council

The **National Academy of Sciences** is a private, nonprofit, self-perpetuating society of distinguished scholars engaged in scientific and engineering research, dedicated to the furtherance of science and technology and to their use for the general welfare. Upon the authority of the charter granted to it by the Congress in 1863, the Academy has a mandate that requires it to advise the federal government on scientific and technical matters. Dr. Bruce M. Alberts is president of the National Academy of Sciences.

The **National Academy of Engineering** was established in 1964, under the charter of the National Academy of Sciences, as a parallel organization of outstanding engineers. It is autonomous in its administration and in the selection of its members, sharing with the National Academy of Sciences the responsibility for advising the federal government. The National Academy of Engineering also sponsors engineering programs aimed at meeting national needs, encourages education and research, and recognizes the superior achievements of engineers. Dr. William A. Wulf is president of the National Academy of Engineering.

The **Institute of Medicine** was established in 1970 by the National Academy of Sciences to secure the services of eminent members of appropriate professions in the examination of policy matters pertaining to the health of the public. The Institute acts under the responsibility given to the National Academy of Sciences by its congressional charter to be an adviser to the federal government and, upon its own initiative, to identify issues of medical care, research, and education. Dr. Kenneth I. Shine is president of the Institute of Medicine.

The **National Research Council** was organized by the National Academy of Sciences in 1916 to associate the broad community of science and technology with the Academy's purposes of furthering knowledge and advising the federal government. Functioning in accordance with general policies determined by the Academy, the Council has become the principal operating agency of both the National Academy of Sciences and the National Academy of Engineering in providing services to the government, the public, and the scientific and engineering communities. The Council is administered jointly by both Academies and the Institute of Medicine. Dr. Bruce M. Alberts and Dr. William A. Wulf are chairman and vice chairman, respectively, of the National Research Council.

ACKNOWLEDGMENTS

Our chief debt as authors of this book is to its predecessor: the 1999 Institute of Medicine report, *Marijuana and Medicine: Assessing the Science Base*. Because this landmark study provided the foundation—indeed, the *raison d'etre*—for our own efforts, we must begin by acknowledging the many contributors who made *Marijuana and Medicine* an authoritative document, and one worthy of popularization.

We are also indebted to many people who helped us adapt the Institute of Medicine study for lay readers. A variety of experts contributed supplemental information and answered questions raised in the original report. They include Roger Anderson, Daniel Brookoff, Daniel Nixon, and Andrew Watry, who provided perspectives on patient experiences during clinical trials of medical marijuana and Marinol®. Thanks also to Sue Rusche and Eric Voth for directing us toward these sources. Others responded to many requests for updated information about policy changes and plans for new clinical trials. They include Steve Gust, Tony Moffet, and Roger Pertwee.

For our chapter on medical marijuana and the law, a subject only briefly mentioned in *Marijuana and Medicine*, we received abundant support and advice from Richard Bonnie and Eve Goldstein. Chuck Thomas, Dale Gieringer, and Scott Imler provided prompt, detailed, and thoughtful answers to our questions regarding cannabis buyer's clubs.

This book relies on the original Institute of Medicine report, which was very much a team effort, and we continue to be indebted to the excellent work of Deborah Yarnell and Amelia Mathis. It was first conceived of by Kenneth Shine, President of the Institute of Medicine, Karen Hein, who was Executive Director at the time, and Stephen Mautner, Executive Editor of the National Academy Press. We thank them for their sustained support and enthusiasm for the project. The Robert Wood Johnson Foundation provided financial support for the project.

This book has been reviewed in draft form by individuals chosen for their diverse perspectives and technical expertise, in accordance with procedures approved by the National Research Council's Report Review Committee. The purpose of this independent review is to provide candid and critical comments that will assist the Institute of Medicine in making its publications as sound as possible and to ensure that they meet institutional standards for objectivity and evidence. The authors wish to thank the following individuals for their participation in the review of this report: Jack D. Barchas, Weill Medical College of Cornell University, Ithaca, New York; John A. Benson, Jr., Oregon Health Sciences University School of Medicine, Portland; Richard J. Bonnie, University of Virginia, Charlottesville; Catherine A. Warren, North Carolina State University, Raleigh; Stanley J. Watson, Jr., University of Michigan, Ann Arbor; and Hallie Wilfert, Institute of Medicine, Washington, D.C.

While the individuals listed above have provided constructive comments and suggestions, it must be emphasized that responsibility for the final content of this report rests entirely with the authors and the Institute of Medicine.

We owe our editor Stephen Mautner enormous gratitude, most notably for his monumental patience when our initially straightforward project became a lengthy, complicated one. Also, since he was involved in this project from its earliest beginnings, we thank him for bringing us together as well as for keeping us there.

Alison wishes to thank the many people whose hard work and kindness enabled her to complete this book, despite complications of pregnancy and its joyous, but chaotic, aftermath. They include the high-risk maternity and NICU nursing staff at

Christiana Hospital and her "extended family" at Wilmington Montessori School. Janet Joy inspired me with her scientific expertise and—sometimes more importantly—buoyed me with her infectious sense of humor. Words cannot express my gratitude for the limitless help and support I received during this adventure from my husband, Tony Kinney, and my mother, Marjorie Mack.

Janet wishes to thank John Benson and Stan Watson, Principal Investigators of the original report. They were a "dream team"—grouchy when necessary, unfailingly supportive, and as intellectually honest as they were demanding. Alison Mack was the last addition to the dream team. She managed to keep this project, which grew larger than either of us envisioned, moving forward in the face of great difficulty.

Alison Mack
Janet Joy

CONTENTS

PREFACE

In recent years there has been unprecedented interest in whether marijuana or its constituent compounds should be used as medicine. Since 1996 voters in eight states have approved the medical use of marijuana. These state ballot initiatives, and the wider discussion they spawned about appropriate national policies regulating marijuana, have been sharply divisive. Advocates of personal choice with a growing distrust of scientific medicine seek alternatives congruent with their values about health and life. Others dismiss medical marijuana as a subterfuge enabling liberalization, which they fear will spread the plague of drug abuse. Medical use might legitimize the drug as safe and effective and justify experimentation by susceptible young people. Both sides cite scientific evidence to support their views.

The director of the White House Office of National Drug Control Policy (ONDCP) asked the Institute of Medicine (IOM) to review the evidence for the potential benefits and risks associated with the use of marijuana. The IOM is a non-governmental, apolitical, non-profit organization of scientists whose independence and objectivity lend credibility to its studies and recommendations. The report of the 18-month IOM study was first released to both the ONDCP and the public in March 1999.

The study team sought and obtained opinions from both sides of the debate, learned of many personal experiences from public hearings, cannabis clubs, and correspondence; anecdotes and opinions were carefully weighed. The team was also informed by dozens of consultant scientists, particularly those engaged in the striking recent advances in the molecular biology, pharmacology, neurochemistry, and social sciences. Exhaustive literature searches led to the citation of over 500 selected scientific papers related to the broad scope of the study. There is remarkable consensus about the fast-moving science that suggests the potential of cannabinoid drugs for medical use. There are far less convincing data about proven medical benefits.

This new book is faithful in every way to the original IOM report. The co-investigators reviewed the manuscript in detail. Symptoms if not diseases can be relieved, but for most patients there are more effective approved medicines today. On the other hand, the basic science suggests potential benefits of certain cannabinoids, delivered without the hazards of smoking, in combination with other drugs using different receptor systems in the brain. The report recommends continued research to elaborate that potentials and thorough epidemiological studies to define suspected risks such as lung cancer from smoking marijuana. Review of the science behind marijuana and cannabinoid convinces us that the often emotional debate so far has been miscast. Medical use of potent, controlled psychoactive drugs has not led to their abuse. Rather than focusing on drug control policy, the medical marijuana debate should really be about the promise of future drug development. We hope this book will further such understanding.

John A. Benson, Jr., M.D.
Stanley J. Watson, Jr., M.D., Ph.D.

MARIJUANA AS MEDICINE?

I

MARIJUANA, MEDICINE, AND SCIENCE

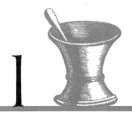

INTRODUCTION

There are many reasons for wanting to understand what science has so far revealed—and what remains un-known—about marijuana's medical potential. Can marijuana really help people with AIDS (acquired immune deficiency syndrome), cancer, glaucoma, multiple sclerosis, or any of several other conditions it is purported to relieve? How does marijuana affect the human body? Could the potential benefits of legalizing marijuana for medicinal use possibly outweigh the risk of encouraging drug abuse? All of these questions remain to be answered completely, but over the past two decades scientists have made significant progress in revealing how chemicals in marijuana act on the body. Researchers have also studied how marijuana use affects individuals and society as a whole.

Unfortunately, much of what scientists have learned about the medical use of marijuana has been obscured by highly polarized debate over the drug's legal status. At times advocates for medical marijuana have appeared to be discussing a different drug than their opponents. Consider the following statements:

> There are over ten thousand documented studies available that confirm the harmful physical and psychological effects of . . . marijuana.
>
> —from the California Narcotic Officers' Association
> *Marijuana is NOT a Medicine*, Santa Clarita, CA (1996), p. 2.

> The cannabis plant (marijuana) . . . [has] therapeutic benefits and
> could ease the suffering of millions of persons with various illnesses
> such as AIDS, cancer, glaucoma, multiple sclerosis, spinal cord in-
> juries, seizure disorders, chronic pain, and other maladies.
> —from the editor's introduction to *Cannabis in Medical Practice,*
> by Mary Lynn Mathre, R.N.

Conflicts regarding the legitimacy of medical marijuana use extend even to the level of state versus federal law. Between 1996 and 1999, voters in eight states (Alaska, Arizona, California, Colorado, Maine, Nevada, Oregon, and Washington) and the District of Columbia* registered their support for the prescription of marijuana by physicians, defying the policies of the federal government and the convictions of many of its leaders.

Prior to the 1998 election, former Presidents Ford, Carter, and Bush released a statement urging voters to reject state medical marijuana initiatives because they circumvented the standard process by which the Food and Drug Administration (FDA) tests medicines for safety and effectiveness. "Compassionate medicine," these leaders insisted, "must be based on science, not political appeals." Nevertheless, medical marijuana initiatives proceeded to pass in every state in which they appeared on the ballot.

Both those who advocate and those who oppose the medical use of marijuana claim to have science on their side. Each camp selectively cites research that supports its position, and each occasionally misrepresents study findings. Unfortunately, these skewed interpretations have frequently served as the main source of scientific information on the subject. Until now it has been difficult for people other than scientists to find unbiased answers to questions about the medical use of marijuana—questions that have often drawn conflicting responses from either side of the debate.

---

*The Colorado vote was later disallowed after a court determined that the petition to place the initiative on the ballot did not have enough valid signatures. Congress has prohibited the counting of actual ballots in the District of Columbia referendum, but exit polls indicated that a majority of voters approved the measure. Nevada voters must reapprove their proposal in the year 2000 before it becomes law.

But the public controversy over the medical use of marijuana does not reflect scientific controversy. Scientists who study marijuana and its effects on the human body largely agree about the risks posed by its use as well as the potential benefits it may provide. That is what researchers at the Institute of Medicine (IOM) learned when they undertook the study on which this book is based.

The goal of the study, performed at the request of the White House Office of National Drug Control Policy, was to conduct a critical review of all scientific evidence pertaining to the medical use of marijuana and its chemical components. For more than a year, researchers from the IOM—an arm of the National Academy of Sciences, which acts as an independent adviser to the federal government—compiled and assessed a broad range of information on the subject. One of us (Janet E. Joy) coordinated the IOM study. John A. Benson, Jr., dean and professor of medicine emeritus from the Oregon Health Sciences University School of Medicine and Stanley J. Watson, Jr., codirector and research scientist at the University of Michigan's Health Research Institute in Ann Arbor, served as its chief investigators. Nine other medical scientists with expertise concerning the medical use of marijuana served as technical advisers throughout the project.

In the course of its work, the study team examined research on how marijuana exerts its effects in the body and its ability to treat a wide variety of medical conditions. Team members compared the effectiveness of using marijuana versus approved medicines to treat numerous specific disorders. They also evaluated the effects of chronic marijuana use on physical and mental health as well as its possible role as a "gateway" drug to cocaine, heroin, and other illicit drugs.

To gather this information, the researchers analyzed scientific publications, consulted extensively with biomedical and social scientists, and conducted public scientific workshops. They also visited four so-called cannabis buyers' clubs and two HIV-AIDS clinics. Organizations and individuals were encouraged to express their views on the medical use of marijuana at the public workshops as well as via the Internet, by mail, and by telephone. The team's draft report was reviewed and critiqued anonymously by more than a dozen experts, whose comments were addressed in preparing the final version of the document. Entitled *Marijuana and Medicine: Assessing the Science Base*, the final report was released in March 1999. The report was subsequently published as a clothbound book by the National Academy Press; it can also be viewed on the Press's web site.

At the time of its release, the study received considerable attention from the news media. For example, the next week more than 50 U.S. newspapers carried stories on the study. While many of the articles reflected the balanced nature of the report's findings, most of the headlines—which tend to stick in readers' minds—gave the impression that the IOM had fully endorsed the medical use of marijuana. Scores of editorials followed suit, including several expressing uncritical acceptance of marijuana as a medicine.

In fact, the IOM researchers found little reason to recommend crude marijuana as a medicine, particularly when smoked, but they did conclude that active ingredients in marijuana could be developed into a variety of promising pharmaceuticals. Responding to the report's call for clinical trials on such marijuana-based medications, the National Institutes of Health and the Canadian equivalent of that agency, Health Canada, subsequently announced new policies intended to encourage medical research on marijuana (see Chapter 11).

While the IOM report was directed at policymakers, the purpose of this book is to present the main findings of that study for use by anyone who wants unbiased, scientifically sound medical information on marijuana. To adapt the IOM's publication for a general audience, considerable technical detail has been removed and in-depth explanations added of several key studies reviewed in the original report. For studies discussed in detail, references are provided in the form of footnotes. When the results of a group of studies are summarized, readers are referred to the relevant pages of the IOM report for more information and complete references. In a few instances, where more recent survey data became available after the IOM report was published, the most current information is used.

This book is divided into three parts, each of which offers a different perspective on marijuana as medicine. Along with this introduction, Chapters 2 and 3 lay out the scientific and historical foundation of current knowledge on the potential benefits and dangers of marijuana-based medicines. The second section—Chapters 4 through 9—focuses on specific diseases, including cancer, AIDS, glaucoma, and a variety of movement and neurological disorders. In each case, the current state of knowledge regarding marijuana's effectiveness in treating symptoms of specific disorders is described and compared with conventional therapies. We explain why some marijuana-related studies that may seem convincing are actually inconclusive and what evidence is needed to support various claims about marijuana's harms or benefits. Finally, although this is primarily a book about science, two chapters in Part III are devoted to related issues: the economic prospects for developing pharmaceuticals from marijuana (Chapter 10) and the complex legal environment surrounding the medical use of marijuana (Chapter 11). Much of the information that is included about the legal status of marijuana did not appear in the IOM report but was added here to place the science of medical marijuana in a broader social context.

In addition to providing a critical and up-to-date summary of scientific knowledge that pertains to the medical use of whole marijuana, chemicals derived from the marijuana plant are also discussed, as well as synthetic compounds that represent "improved" versions of marijuana derivatives. This information can help readers evaluate future research news and participate in the ongoing public discussion of medical marijuana.

At the same time, it is important to recognize that science is but one aspect of the medical marijuana controversy. Ultimately, drug laws must address moral, social, and political concerns as well as science and medicine. Although we present scientific evidence related to the social impact of medical marijuana, the intent is not to prescribe policy but to encourage continued debate based on a firm understanding of scientific knowledge. As you read, please bear this in mind, along with the following caveats:

- Neither this book, nor the IOM study on which it is based, is intended to promote specific social policies. Both were designed to provide an objective scientific analysis of marijuana's current and potential usefulness in treating a variety of symptoms.
- In no way do we wish to suggest that patients should, un-

der any circumstance, medicate themselves with marijuana, an illegal drug.

• The medical information in this book is not intended to substitute for the advice of a physician or other health care professional.

Now that you know where this book came from and where it's going, we offer a few guideposts to aid your journey through it. Because the following key concepts underlie our discussion of medical marijuana, familiarizing yourself with them will help you make the most of your reading.

Marijuana contains a complex mixture of chemicals. Marijuana leaves or flower tops can be smoked, eaten, or drunk as a tea (see Figure 1.1). People who use marijuana in these ways expose themselves to the complex mixture of chemical compounds present in the plant. One of these chemicals, tetrahydrocannabinol (THC), is the main cause of the marijuana "high." Thus, the effects of marijuana on the body include those of THC, but not all of marijuana's effects are necessarily due to THC alone.

According to federal law, marijuana belongs to a category of substances that have a high potential for abuse and no accepted medical use. Other drugs in this category include LSD (lysergic acid diethylamide) and heroin. By contrast, doctors can legally prescribe THC, in the form of the medicine Marinol (a brand name for a specific formulation of the generic drug dronabinol), under highly regulated conditions. Dronabinol, the "synthetic" THC in Marinol, is identical in every way to the "natural" THC in marijuana.

The FDA has approved Marinol for the treatment of nausea and vomiting associated with cancer chemotherapy and also to counteract weight loss in AIDS patients. Currently classified with controlled substances such as anabolic steroids, Marinol was moved from a more restrictive category, which included cocaine and morphine, in July 1999.

Some of the medical studies discussed in later chapters deal with the effects of marijuana, while others focus on specific chemicals present in the marijuana plant. This distinction should be kept in mind when considering the results of these studies. The psychoactive chemicals in marijuana are members of a family of mol-

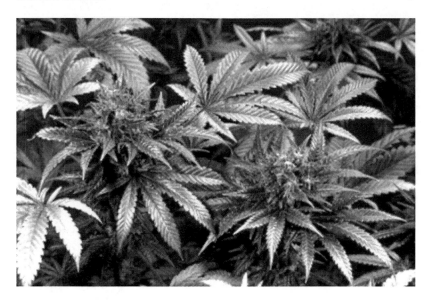

FIGURE 1.1 Leaves and flower tops of female marijuana plants. (Photo by André Grossman.)

ecules known as *cannabinoids*, derived from the plant's scientific name, *Cannabis sativa*. Most cannabinoids are closely related to THC. Scientists also refer to chemicals that are not found in marijuana but that resemble THC either in their chemical structure or the way they affect the body as cannabinoids.

Occasionally, we also refer to "marijuana-based medicines." These encompass the entire spectrum of potential medications derived from marijuana, from whole-plant remedies to extracts to individual cannabinoids, both natural and synthetic.

Marijuana is not a modern medicine. Although people have used marijuana for centuries to soothe a variety of ills, it cannot be considered a medicine in the same sense as, for example, aspirin. Aspirin's chemical cousin, found in willow bark, was long used as a folk remedy for pain. But unlike marijuana, aspirin has been proven safe and effective through rigorous testing. Aspirin tablets contain a pure measured dose of medicine, so they can be relied on to give consistent and predictable results.

By contrast, two identical-looking marijuana cigarettes could produce quite different effects, even if smoked by the same person. If one of the cigarettes were made mostly from leaves and the other from flower tops, for instance, they would probably contain different amounts of active chemicals. Growing conditions also affect marijuana's potency, which can vary greatly from region to region and even from season to season in the same place. This variability makes marijuana at best a crude remedy, more akin to herbal supplements such as St. John's wort or ginkgo than to conventional medications.

To date, few herbal supplements have been tested for safety and efficacy in the United States, nor are such products subject to mandatory quality controls. Yet despite these drawbacks, increasing numbers of consumers are using herbal treatments, prompted by their desire for "natural" alternatives to man-made medicines. However, another way to view herbal remedies is to recognize that if they are effective, they contain specific active ingredients. Willow bark contains a pain-relieving compound; marijuana contains cannabinoids such as THC, which lessens nausea. Once identified, chemists can duplicate active compounds in the laboratory. Scientists can also use natural compounds as a basis for creating new medicines. By introducing subtle structural changes in natural molecules, chemists have produced drugs that are more effective and easier to administer and that have fewer side effects than their natural counterparts. So far, a few such analogs or derivatives of cannabinoids are known to exist; others are currently under investigation.

Marijuana used as medicine is not a recreational drug. People who use marijuana solely as a medication do so in order to relieve specific symptoms of AIDS, cancer, multiple sclerosis, and other debilitating conditions. Some do so under the advice or consent of doctors after conventional treatments have failed to help them. In mentioning medical marijuana users, we are referring to people who smoke or eat marijuana exclusively as a treatment for medical symptoms. The fact that many such patients may have prior recreational experience with the drug does not mean that they are using illness as an excuse to get high, although it is possible that some patients might do so. Surveys of marijuana buyers' clubs indicate that most of their members do, in fact, have serious medical conditions.

Medical marijuana users tend to come from different segments of the population than recreational users. In the United States recreational marijuana use is most prevalent among 18 to 25 year olds and declines sharply after age 34. By contrast, reports on medical marijuana users indicate that most are over 35, as are typical consumers of herbal medicine and other alternative therapies. Most tend to suffer from chronic illnesses or pain that defy conventional treatments.

Medical marijuana advocates assert that patients usually obtain relief with smaller doses of the drug than would be used recreationally and that they rarely feel high when treating their symptoms with marijuana; however, no objective study has tested this claim. As discussed in detail in Chapter 3, marijuana and its constituent chemicals can produce both physical and psychological dependence. These risks must be taken into account if marijuana or cannabinoids are to be used as medicines.

Many effective medicines have side effects. The fact that marijuana affects the human body adversely does not preclude its use as a source of useful medicines. Many legitimate drugs—including opiates, chemotherapy agents, and steroids—have side effects ranging from the dangerous to the merely unpleasant. When used carefully, though, the benefits of these medications far outweigh their drawbacks. Patients may also develop tolerance, dependence, and withdrawal—conditions associated with marijuana use—when taking proper doses of several commonly prescribed medications. For example, the correct use of some prescription medicines for pain, anxiety, and even hypertension normally produces tolerance and some physiological dependence.

As researchers learn more about the chemicals present in marijuana and their effects on the body, it may be possible to identify beneficial compounds and separate them from harmful substances in the plant. Finding a rapid way to deliver cannabinoids to the body, other than smoking, could lessen some of marijuana's worst side effects. It may also be possible to reduce the adverse effects of specific cannabinoids through chemical modification, as previously noted.

Marijuana's effects vary with different delivery methods. Traditionally, medicinal marijuana has not been smoked but rather swallowed in the form of an extract or applied to the underside of the tongue in the form of an alcohol-based tincture. Although the latter method allows the THC to pass directly into the bloodstream, it is far less efficient than smoking. When swallowed, drugs pass through the stomach, intestine, and liver before entering the bloodstream, so they act slowly. This is especially true of the main active ingredient in marijuana. Because THC is barely soluble in water, the body absorbs only a small fraction of the available drug when it is swallowed.

The same is true of Marinol, which is simply THC in capsule form. Marijuana smoke, on the other hand, efficiently delivers THC into the bloodstream via the lungs. Inhaled THC takes effect quickly, allowing patients to use just enough to relieve their symptoms; it is not so easy to fine-tune the dose of oral medications. For this reason, pharmaceutical firms are investigating the use of smokeless inhalers and nasal sprays to deliver THC and possibly other cannabinoids.

2

CAN MARIJUANA HELP?

Current knowledge about marijuana's effects derives from three main sources: personal and historical accounts of its use, a limited number of clinical studies, and basic scientific research on marijuana and its constituent compounds. Clinical studies, which are discussed in Part II of this book, measure the overall effects of drugs on human subjects. Basic research, on the other hand, examines the specific effects of drugs on cells and on the biochemical reactions that take place within them. Basic studies have been conducted to characterize the chemicals found in marijuana, their interactions with molecules and cells in the human body, and their effects on experimental animals.

The most readily available information on medical marijuana can be found in historical documents—some more than a thousand years old—as well in the personal stories of people who have taken the drug to relieve medical symptoms. In addition to such anecdotes, scientific research recently has begun to reveal clues to marijuana's potential benefits. This chapter presents a broad summary of both anecdotal and basic scientific evidence of marijuana's promise as a source of medicine.

A BRIEF HISTORY OF MEDICAL MARIJUANA

The marijuana plant—also known as hemp and cannabis—has been used throughout agricultural history as a source of in-

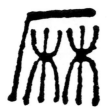

FIGURE 2.1 The Chinese ideogram for marijuana ("ma") shows two plants, male and female, under a drying shed. (Drawing from *Cannabis in Medical Practice*, M. L. Mathre, ed., McFarland and Company, Inc., 1997, p. 36.)

toxicant, medicine, and fiber. The earliest known descriptions of marijuana appear in the ancient writings and folklore of India and China, where historians believe it was first used as a ritual intoxicant. Eventually, marijuana was put to common use in folk medicine, usually in the form of a tea or edible extract. The medicinal use of smoked marijuana is largely a recent phenomenon.[1]

According to Chinese legend, the emperor Shen Nung (circa 2700 B.C.; also known as Chen Nung) discovered marijuana's healing properties as well as those of two other mainstays of Chinese herbal medicine, ginseng and ephedra. In a compendium of drug recipes compiled in 1 A.D., based on traditions from the time of Shen Nung, marijuana is depicted as an ideogram of plants drying in a shed (see Figure 2.1). This ancient text, which is considered to be the world's oldest pharmacopoeia, recommends marijuana for more than 100 ailments, including gout, rheumatism, malaria, and absentmindedness. Centuries later a Chinese medical text (1578 A.D.) described the use of marijuana to treat vomiting, parasitic infections, and hemorrhage. Marijuana continues to be used in China as a folk remedy for diarrhea and dysentery and to stimulate the appetite.[2]

In India, marijuana has been associated with magic and religion—as well as healing—for thousands of years. Practitioners of traditional Ayurvedic medicine still prescribe marijuana to promote sleep, appetite, and digestion as well as to relieve pain; it is also considered an aphrodisiac and intoxicant.

By contrast, ancient Greek and Roman physicians cautioned that excess use of marijuana could dampen sexual performance.[3] Despite this drawback, Galen (2 A.D.) and Pliny the Elder (circa 25 A.D.) as well as Discorides—a doctor in the army of the Roman emperor Nero (1 A.D.)—recommended marijuana as a treatment for a variety of ailments, including earache.

Marijuana's double nature—harmful intoxicant versus beneficial medicine—was debated at least as early as the fifteenth century. At that time, Muslim theologians were faced with the question of whether hashish (a potent drug made from marijuana resin) should be treated like alcohol, which is specifically forbidden by the Koran. In solving this dilemma the scholars distinguished between the use of hashish as an intoxicant, for which they recommended punishment by brutal whipping, and its permissible use as a medicine.[4]

Muslims also invented techniques to manufacture paper from hemp fibers, a process that was introduced to Europe during the twelfth century. Hemp remained an important component of most paper products until the mid-nineteenth century, when it was replaced by wood pulp. Arab traders are also thought to have conveyed their knowledge of hemp's medicinal properties to Africa during medieval times. There marijuana came to be widely used to treat a variety of ailments, including snakebite, labor pains, malaria, and dysentery.[5]

By contrast, there is little evidence that marijuana was used as a medicine in medieval Europe. During the Renaissance, reports from explorers in Asia, Africa, and the Middle East piqued the interest of European herbalists, who also consulted the writings of Galen, Pliny, and other ancient physicians. Nevertheless, medical marijuana continued to be a rarity in the West.[6] Meanwhile, demand for hemp fibers as a material for making rope and textiles—especially canvas for sails—grew so strong that by the sixteenth century European nations commanded their colonies to grow the crop. There is, however, no evidence that colonists used the plant for anything but its fiber. It was not until the mid-nineteenth century that Western medicine "discovered" marijuana (see Figure 2.2).[7]

It was an Irish doctor, William O'Shaughnessy, who was largely responsible for acquainting his Western colleagues with marijuana's healing properties. O'Shaughnessy learned of the herb as a professor at the Medical College of Calcutta. In the 1830s, he created marijuana preparations and tested their effects on animals; convinced that they were safe, he began administering them to patients as a treatment for pain and muscle spasms. He also

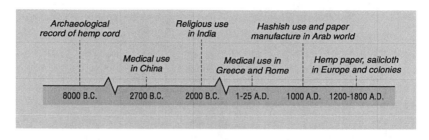

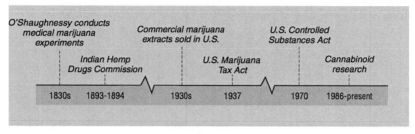

FIGURE 2.2 Medical marijuana timelines.

reported success in using marijuana to treat the often-fatal vomiting and diarrhea associated with cholera.[8]

O'Shaughnessy's discoveries fascinated physicians in Europe and America, provoking a flurry of Western research on medical marijuana that lasted well into the twentieth century. Hundreds of Indian and Western doctors described marijuana's medical benefits before the Indian Hemp Drugs Commission, convened by the British in 1893-1894. They told of treating cramps, headache, asthma, diabetes, impotence, acute and chronic pain, fever, appetite loss, and scores of other conditions with the plant. On the basis of this testimony, members of the commission concluded that marijuana represented one of the most important drugs in the Indian pharmacopoeia and that "moderate use of hemp drugs is practically attended by no evil results at all." Thus, the commission recommended against marijuana's prohibition, despite acknowledging the problems posed by its abuse as an intoxicant.[9]

At the first American conference on the clinical use of marijuana, held by the Ohio State Medical Society in 1860, physicians reported success in using marijuana to treat chronic cough, gonorrhea, pain, and a variety of other conditions. As demand for marijuana-based medications accelerated, pharmaceutical firms attempted to produce consistently potent and reliable drugs from hemp. By the 1930s at least two American companies—Parke-Davis and Eli Lilly—were selling standardized extracts of marijuana for use as an analgesic, an antispasmodic and sedative (see Figure 2.3). Another manufacturer, Grimault & Company, marketed marijuana cigarettes as a remedy for asthma.[10]

But shortly after pure marijuana preparations became available, more effective synthetic drugs such as aspirin and barbiturates began replacing herbal remedies. Meanwhile, recreational marijuana smoking became popular among jazz-age musicians and artists in the United States and with it claims that it caused crime, mental illness, and even death. Against the advice of the American Medical Association, the U.S. Congress passed the Marijuana Tax Act of 1937, which imposed tough restrictions on marijuana sales and prescription. As a result, most pharmaceutical companies ceased producing marijuana-based drugs. In 1942 marijuana was removed from the *United States Pharmacopoeia* (USP) on the grounds that it was a harmful and addictive drug.[11]

Interestingly, marijuana is not the only drug that has progressed, over the ages, from folk medicine to conventional treatment to highly regulated substance of abuse. The narcotic opium, produced from the dried resin of immature poppy flowers, has been used as a pain remedy for nearly 2,000 years. Taken by mouth, its effects are too weak to encourage abuse. But after smoking opium—which rapidly induces an intense "high"—became popular in seventeenth-century China, many people became addicted to the drug.

Opium soon made its way into Europe and North America, where it was both used as a painkiller and abused by addicts. The pure compound morphine, first isolated from opium in the early eighteenth century, gained wide use as an analgesic, particularly during surgery. Heroin, a chemical derivative of morphine, and codeine, another natural opiate, also were developed as painkillers. As with cannabinoids, the human body produces its own version of opiates, known as endorphins. These compounds interact with nerve cells in the same way as their plant-derived relatives, with similarly soothing results.

Although natural and synthetic opiates are among the most

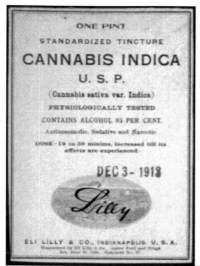

FIGURE 2.3 Labels from patent medicines that contained marijuana. (Courtesy of Eli Lilly and Company Archives.)

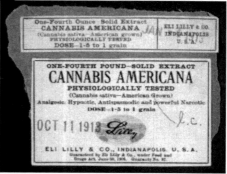

effective pain relievers, they are highly regulated due to their great potential for abuse. As a result, many doctors hesitate to prescribe opiate medications except in extreme cases. Nevertheless, opiate abuse is so widespread that the illegal demand for opium far exceeds legitimate medicinal sales of the drug.[12]

More than a century after opium abuse spread across the globe, marijuana gained worldwide popularity as a recreational drug. By the 1960s, marijuana use had become widespread, and in 1970, the U.S. government passed the landmark Controlled Substances Act. This law organized all drugs with abuse potential into five schedules, according to three criteria: the likelihood that the drug would be abused, its medical usefulness, and the physical and psychological consequences of its abuse. Marijuana, along with LSD and heroin, was placed in Schedule I, the most restrictive category. Schedule I substances are considered to have no medical use and a high potential for abuse.

That classification continues to be challenged by the National Organization for the Reform of Marijuana Laws and medical marijuana advocates. In addition, since passage of the federal Controlled Substances Act, several states have placed marijuana in a less restrictive category in their own controlled substance laws. In the 1970s and 1980s several states even supported limited clinical studies on medical marijuana. Voters in several states have passed referenda intended to permit marijuana use for medical purposes (see Chapter 11).

USERS' VIEWS

Despite its illegality, millions of Americans use marijuana regularly. A small minority—most of whom had previously used the drug recreationally—smoke or eat it to relieve various medical symptoms. In three public hearings held by the IOM as part of its study of medical marijuana, 43 such patients came forward to relate their experiences (see Figure 2.4); the research team also

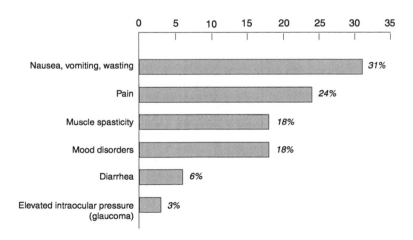

FIGURE 2.4 Reported medical uses of marijuana. Frequency of symptoms among 43 patients who spoke at the IOM's public workshops. Twenty of these patients reported using marijuana to relieve more than one symptom.

spoke with several dozen members of three medical marijuana buyers' clubs in California. Patients described using marijuana to treat AIDS wasting, spasticity from multiple sclerosis, depression, chronic pain, chemotherapy-induced nausea, and other symptoms. Similar accounts of medical marijuana use in treating an even broader range of conditions appear in *Marihuana: The Forbidden Medicine*, by Lester Grinspoon and James Bakalar.[13]

AIDS was the predominant disorder described by medical marijuana users who told their stories to the IOM study team. Many such speakers said they used marijuana to combat wasting and to reduce the side effects of other medications. A typical account follows, presented by a 35-year-old Florida writer who discovered he was HIV-positive in 1987.

> Skin rashes, dry mouth, foul metallic aftertaste, numbness of the face, swelling of the limbs, fever spikes, headaches, dizziness, anemia, clinical depression, neuropathy so crippling that I could not type, so painful that the bed sheets felt like sandpaper, nausea so severe that I sometimes had to leave the dinner table to vomit, and diarrhea so unpredictable that I dared not leave the house without diapers.
>
> These are some of the horrors that I endured in the last 10 years during my fight for life against HIV [human immunodeficiency virus]. But these ravages were not caused by HIV itself, or by any of the opportunistic infections that mark the steady progression of AIDS. Each of these nightmares was a side effect of one of the hundreds of medications I have taken to fight one infection after another on my way to a seemingly early grave.
>
> Had you known me three years ago you would not recognize me now. After years of final-stage AIDS, I had wasted to 130 pounds. The purple Kaposi's sarcoma lesions were spreading. The dark circles under my eyes told of sleepless nights and half-waking days. I knew that I was dying.
>
> But still I was fortunate because along the way I rediscovered the ancient understanding of marijuana's medicinal benefit. So I smoked pot. Every day. The pot calmed my stomach against handfuls of pills. The pot made me hungry so that I could eat without a tube. The pot eased the crippling neural side effects so that I could dial the phone by myself. The pot calmed my soul and allowed me to accept that I would probably die soon. Because I smoked pot, I lived long enough to celebrate my thirty-fifth birthday. I lived to sit on the bus without frightening the passenger beside me.

Even at this stage of my recovery, I take a handful of pills almost every day, and will probably continue to do so for the rest of my life. While I am grateful for the life-saving protease inhibitor therapies, they bring with them a host of adverse reactions and undesirable side effects. Smoking marijuana relieves many of these side effects.

I sit here, I believe, as living proof that marijuana can have a beneficial effect in staving off wasting. I figured that every pound of body weight I could maintain, that was another day that I could live in hopes that some effective therapy would emerge.

Others described how marijuana helped them cope with nausea and vomiting during chemotherapy—symptoms that defied otherwise effective treatments:

I guess I am one of the luckier people who will be appearing before you today because my medical problem was testicular cancer. People do die of testicular cancer, but the cure rates are very high, 90 percent or over. There is one form of chemotherapy that seems to work.

Now the down side of the chemotherapy—it is one of the rougher [treatments]. The drug is called cisplatin, and it is known for the nausea that it induces. The legal antinausea drugs were pretty good. For my first two courses of chemotherapy I did not have a problem with nausea. However, by the end of the second course, I could tell that the effect of the Zofran [that I had been given to control my nausea] was wearing off. So, for my third and fourth courses of chemotherapy, I smoked marijuana.

None of my doctors and nurses discouraged me from doing this. I was being treated at NYU Medical Center in New York, and I went for a consultation at Memorial Sloan-Kettering. So I was getting the best possible care.

I found that when I smoked marijuana the effect came . . . in a couple of minutes, and the symptoms of nausea would go away. Interestingly, I did not consider taking Marinol [oral dronabinol, equivalent to THC], and my doctor did not recommend that I try [it]. What I was dealing with was nausea, and it didn't seem to me that taking a pill was a very intelligent or effective way to combat nausea.

I didn't find that it [smoking marijuana] impeded my work [the speaker is a well-known conservative journalist]. It certainly didn't turn me into a drug addict. I had smoked maybe a dozen times recreationally in college. I would never touch a joint again unless I got cancer again and I had to take it [to relieve nausea]. The mere thought of smoking something that is associated with the bad experience [of chemotherapy] is very aversive to me.

Similarly, one woman reported that marijuana helped her keep down her migraine medication:

> I started smoking marijuana when I was 19, as a recreational drug. I had no idea of any sort of medical or therapeutic uses whatsoever. Three years before that I had been diagnosed with migraines, and I have suffered [from] them pretty continuously since that time. Right about 1989 or 1990, after I started using marijuana recreationally, a lot more information about marijuana started to become available. At that point I realized that maybe the convergence of my recreational use and my medical condition might be possible.
>
> My doctor had prescribed a [migraine] medicine called Ergomar. It had really bad effects. The headache might go away or it might not. Either way I would definitely throw up if I took the medicine. [I switched to] Imitrex after that. Imitrex does work to remove my migraines, and marijuana never has been able to do that. But marijuana relieves my nausea enough that I can keep my pharmaceutical medication down.

Next to AIDS and chemotherapy-induced nausea, pain appears to be the most frequently cited reason for using medical marijuana. Like several individuals who addressed the IOM team, the following man found that marijuana improved the effectiveness of the narcotic medications he was already taking for pain:

> I am a 35-year-old father [and] a United States Air Force disabled veteran. I came to know cannabis in the usual way for a baby boomer, [having] tried it in high school. I left behind cannabis and high school simultaneously in 1981, when I joined the Air Force.
>
> I was serving in the South Pacific . . . when I fell victim to a poorly constructed roadway and crashed my motorcycle. I spent the better part of [the next] two years in and out of the hospital. Now, 14 years, 10 surgeries, and two artificial hips later, I sit before you. You would never guess the extent of my injuries or repairs. I lost parts of my spleen and intestines, and I get . . . awful cramping. I get pain that shoots down to my knee.
>
> I owe a good deal of my excellent recovery to . . . cannabis. My pain medication [Percocet] is less effective without cannabis, and [if I don't use it] I'm forced to take too much narcotic. A few puffs . . . relieve the majority of my stomach spasms, completely eliminate nausea, and allow me to eat an entire meal instead of nibbling.

According to federal law, only eight people in the United States are currently allowed to smoke marijuana for medical reasons. These patients receive marijuana cigarettes prepared by the U.S. government under a Compassionate Use Program, a program that has been closed to new patients since 1992. The surviving participants include this 41-year-old woman who managed her family's men's wear store until she developed multiple sclerosis. She smokes marijuana to relieve several symptoms of multiple sclerosis:

> I was diagnosed with multiple sclerosis in 1988. Prior to that I was an active person with ballet and swimming. I [still] swim each day, and I smoke marijuana. Each month I pick up a can filled with the marijuana cigarettes rolled by the government.
>
> At one time I weighed 85 pounds, and now I weigh 105 pounds. [Before I began smoking marijuana], I could not walk. I did not have an appetite. When I found out that there was a program to get marijuana from the government, I decided that was the answer. I was not a marijuana smoker before that; in fact, I used to consider the people I knew who smoked marijuana as undesirables. Now I myself am an undesirable.
>
> But it works. It takes away the backache. With multiple sclerosis, you can get [muscle] spasms. You may have danced all your life . . . but the MS will take that from you. So I use the swimming pool, and that helps a lot. The kicks are a lot [easier] when I have smoked a marijuana cigarette. Since 1991 I've smoked 10 cigarettes a day. I do not take any other drugs. Marijuana seems to have been my helper.

Another legal marijuana user, this Florida woman described how in 1976 she began using the drug to relieve the symptoms of glaucoma. She received legal permission to use it in 1998:

> When a doctor told me, a year after I had been diagnosed with glaucoma, that I had better start smoking marijuana, I questioned his sanity. He could see that I had already tried . . . Pilocarpine* and a stronger [drug]. Those gave me horrendous headaches, and I could not tolerate them at all. Diamox [another prescription drug for glaucoma] knocked me flat . . . At that point I realized that if I was going to save my sight at the expense of taking the rest of my body down, then it wasn't worth saving.

---

*Pilocarpine and Diamox were among the few drugs available to treat glaucoma in the late 1970s, but they are not popular today because of their side effects. Better glaucoma drugs with fewer side effects are now available.

Compelling though these accounts are, it would be a mistake to use anecdotal evidence to measure marijuana's clinical value. Only thorough clinical studies can compare marijuana's effectiveness with that of existing medications. However, these anecdotal reports do define certain symptoms that warrant clinical investigation: nausea, wasting, pain, muscle spasms, and increased intraocular pressure.

Interestingly, the IOM study team did not receive any direct reports of less than positive experiences with medical marijuana. A few speakers did mention that they knew people whom marijuana had failed to help. Indeed, patients in several clinical studies have occasionally had adverse reactions to smoked marijuana, including anxiety, panic, and paranoia. These short-term effects appear to occur mainly among first-time and older users.[14] It seems doubtful that anyone who reacted this badly to a medication would want to continue taking it, but it is unclear how many potential users of medical marijuana would fall into that category.

No drug—including conventional medications used to treat symptoms for which marijuana has been touted—is free of side effects, however. Medicines represent a balance of risks and benefits. But for marijuana and its constituent chemicals, no one can reliably predict which way that balance will tip for a specific patient.

CANNABINOID SCIENCE

Not long ago most medical treatment was based on anecdotal evidence. Only recently—and only in the world's wealthiest societies—have scientific standards replaced the oral traditions of folk medicine. Although many modern medicines are derived from plants used in traditional healing, they are purified compounds that conform to high standards of safety and efficacy. Thus, before marijuana-based medicines appear on pharmacists' shelves, they must undergo clinical testing to assure that they meet the same exacting standards.

But clinical studies of marijuana are currently difficult to conduct. Scientists interested in pursuing such research face a series of barriers, including limited funding and a daunting thicket of federal and state regulations. No wonder, then, that clinical evidence for marijuana's benefits (discussed in Chapters 4 through 9) is limited indeed.

Yet despite the scarcity of clinical data, several biological studies indicate that marijuana-based drugs could potentially ease a variety of symptoms. These studies fall under the category of basic research and are intended to single out marijuana's many effects and study them individually in order to discover how chemicals in marijuana act on various cells and organ systems in the body. Some of these studies suggest that cannabinoids could be used as the basis for developing new, highly specific medicines with fewer side effects.

Biological studies also offer the possibility of finding new treatments by defining symptom-producing processes that occur in individual cells. Often these mechanisms take the form of chains of biochemical reactions that result in sensations such as pain or nausea—symptoms that might be averted if the chain were interrupted at any point. Thus, for any given symptom the potential exists to discover numerous drugs that reinforce each other's effects, because each affects a unique link in the causal chain. Several basic studies indicate that marijuana acts differently from conventional treatments for a variety of conditions, so it may prove to be a valuable source of auxiliary medicines.

The following sections summarize the findings of several recent studies on the biological effects of marijuana and its chemical components. Readers can find more detailed information (including references) on studies described in these sections in Chapter 2 of the 1999 IOM report, *Marijuana and Medicine: Assessing the Science Base.*

CANNABINOID CHEMISTRY

The active chemicals in marijuana, known as *cannabinoids*, are produced by resin glands on the female plant's leaves, stems, and calyxes, leaflike structures that sheath its small flowers (see Figure 2.5). Marijuana plants are either male or female; the female plant is the source of the drug. Although marijuana flowers themselves do not produce resin, they become a concentrated source of cannabinoids because resin tends to collect in the flower tops. Individual marijuana plants may contain widely differing

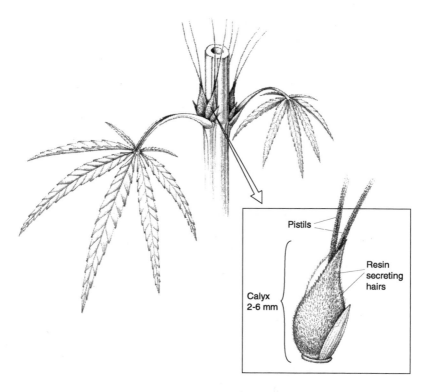

FIGURE 2.5 Female marijuana flowers grow in pairs, close to the main stem at the base of each leaf stem. Each small, petal-less flower is sheathed by a leaf-like structure, the calyx, which is covered with tiny, resin-secreting hairs. The resin contains high concentrations of cannabinoids such as THC, the primary active ingredient in marijuana. (Drawing by Roberto Osti from illustrations in *Marijuana Botany: An Advanced Study: The Propagation and Breeding of Distinctive Cannabis.* Robert Connell Clarke. Berkeley, CA: Ronin Publishing. 1981.)

amounts of specific cannabinoids due to variations in soil, temperature, humidity, and other growth conditions. And because cannabinoids degrade when exposed to high temperatures, moisture, and sunlight, storage conditions strongly affect the cannabinoid content of dried leaves or flower tops.

More than 60 different but closely related cannabinoids have been isolated from marijuana. They are greasy compounds, barely soluble in water, that dissolve readily in oily fluids. The chemical structure of most cannabinoids is similar to THC, the main psychoactive ingredient in marijuana. Although researchers have identified several variants of THC, only the most abundant form, delta-9-THC, has been studied extensively (unless stated otherwise, we use the term THC to refer to this compound). The active ingredient in the prescription medicine Marinol is synthetic THC, which is also known by its generic name, dronabinol. Marinol is used to treat chemotherapy-induced nausea and vomiting as well as AIDS wasting syndrome.

Marijuana plants make THC through a multistep process, much as chemists do when they synthesize THC in the laboratory. A series of assembly steps combine several simple molecules to form a cannabinoid compound called *cannabigerol*. Cannabigerol may be subsequently converted to THC or to another cannabinoid called *cannabidiol*, which may then be modified to produce THC. It in turn may undergo chemical reactions that convert it to yet another cannabinoid, *cannabinol*. Unlike THC, neither cannabigerol, cannabidiol, nor cannabinol is psychoactive. Live marijuana plants and dried plant parts contain all of these cannabinoids as well as others that represent either precursors of THC or modified versions of the THC molecule.

CANNABINOIDS AND THE CELL

Although it has long been observed that marijuana alters thinking and behavior, scientists have only recently begun to learn how chemicals in marijuana act on individual cells, both in the brain and elsewhere in the body. That knowledge is crucial to determining exactly how marijuana and its constituent chemicals affect users.

Recent studies indicate that cannabinoids produce most of their effects by binding to proteins, called receptors, on the surfaces of certain types of cells. Many different types of receptor proteins stud the exterior membranes of the cells throughout the human body. Each receptor recognizes only a few specific molecules, known collectively as ligands. When the appropriate ligand binds to its receptor, it typically sets off a chain of biochemical reactions inside the cell. Many drugs, as well as hormones and neurotransmitters, exert their effects by acting as ligands at different receptors.

The cellular receptors that bind THC and its chemical relatives are known as cannabinoid receptors. All vertebrate animals have similar types of cannabinoid receptors on their cells. So do some invertebrates, such as mollusks and leeches—an indication that the receptors fulfill similar functions in a broad range of animal species. Moreover, it suggests that cannabinoid receptors have existed at least since vertebrates first evolved, more than 500 million years ago.

To date, scientists have identified two main types of cannabinoid receptors, known as CB_1 and CB_2. CB_1 receptors are extraordinarily abundant in the brain; for example, the brain has 10 times as many cannabinoid receptors as "morphine" receptors, which are responsible for the effects of heroin and other opiates (as well as the body's own endorphins). CB_2 receptors, on the other hand, are relatively scarce in the brain but plentiful in the immune system.

Cells bearing cannabinoid receptors respond to ligand binding in a variety of ways. When THC binds CB_1 receptors in some nerve cells, for example, it triggers a cascade of reactions that ultimately slow down nerve impulses. This might slow a person's reaction time enough to make driving hazardous, but the same process could also dull pain signals traveling along those nerves, thereby providing some pain relief. Likewise, when THC binds CB_2 receptors on white blood cells, it may impede their natural response to infection—a bad thing if it lowers a person's resistance to disease but a good thing if it reduces painful inflammation.

Although CB_1 and CB_2 share some structural and functional similarities, the two receptor types are different enough that it may be possible to design ligands that, unlike THC, would act on only one of them. Medicines based on these ligands would be expected to have fewer side effects due to their greater precision. In recent years researchers have discovered several natural ligands that bind only to CB_1 or CB_2; they have also synthesized a few such selective ligands. Although currently used only as research tools, these compounds represent an encouraging start toward developing novel medicines based on cannabinoids.

When researchers identify a receptor in the human body that binds a particular drug, such as THC, they next try to find molecules that naturally interact with the receptor in order to learn more about how the receptor functions and what purposes it serves. Scientists have identified several chemicals produced in the body that act on the cannabinoid receptors, CB_1 and CB_2; however, the physiological functions of these ligands remain unknown. The best studied among these compounds, anandamide (from *ananda*, the Sanskrit word for "bliss"), appears to act throughout the body, especially on the central nervous system. Anandamide is present in high concentrations—along with abundant CB_1 receptors—in areas of the brain that control learning, memory, movement, coordination, and responses to stress. Significant amounts of anandamide are also found in the spleen, which has numerous CB_2 receptors, and the heart.

Compared with THC, anandamide binds cannabinoid receptors weakly. As a result, the reactions that anandamide provokes are probably milder than those triggered by THC. Moreover, enzymes in the body quickly break down anandamide, so its effects are also relatively short lived. Another factor that limits anandamide's activity is a phenomenon known as reuptake, the rapid reabsorption of certain types of neurotransmitters after their release from nerve cells (see Figure 2.6), which protects neighboring nerve cells from over-stimulation. In some cases, this "protection" system can be adjusted to provide a therapeutic benefit. For example, the antidepressant Prozac works by blocking the reuptake of the neurotransmitter serotonin. If researchers found an analogous compound that prevented anandamide reuptake, perhaps it could be used to relieve distressed patients by raising the level of natural cannabinoids in their brains. Such a drug could potentially deliver many of the benefits of THC but with fewer side effects.

In addition to anandamide, researchers have identified several chemicals produced by the human body that bind to cannabinoid receptors, and they are continually finding more. These compounds are thought to perform a broad range of functions in the brain. Over the next few years scientists are likely to learn much more about these naturally occurring endogenous cannabinoids.

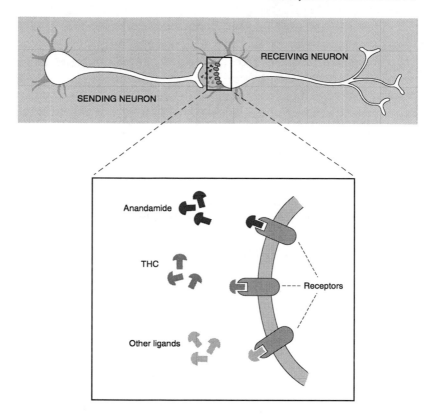

FIGURE 2.6 Signaling between nerve cells. Signal transmission between two neurons (nerve cells) begins as the sending neuron releases chemical messengers called neurotransmitters. Neurotransmitter molecules move across the gap to the receiving neuron, where they are bound by receptors on its surface. Binding may activate the receptor, triggering a chain of events that can alter thought and behavior.

The magnified view shows a variety of ligands binding to different types of receptors present on neurons. Anandamide, which is produced by the body, and THC, the main psychoactive ingredient in marijuana, can function as neurotransmitters. Both compounds bind and activate cannabinoid receptors on nerve cells, much as other neurotransmitters bind and activate their own specific receptors.

Researchers have also noted that cannabinoids can affect the body without binding to receptors. Both THC and cannabidiol have been shown to reduce toxic forms of oxygen that build up in tissues under stress, as do the antioxidant vitamins A and C. Also, because cannabinoids dissolve easily in the fatty membranes enclosing every cell, they may alter membrane function and, along with it, the activity of enzymes and proteins embedded in cell membranes. These properties, too, may prove medically useful.

CANNABINOIDS AND THE NERVOUS SYSTEM

Because cannabinoids and their receptors are naturally present throughout the human body, scientists suspect that the compounds serve a wide variety of physiological functions. That is especially true in the brain and spinal cord, which contain numerous CB_1 receptors. When cannabinoids bind to these receptors, they typically set off a chain reaction that slows the transmission of nerve impulses between cells. That is not always the case, however; in other nerve cells, CB_1 receptors are arranged in such a way that they speed the delivery of messages along neural pathways.

The largest populations of CB_1 receptors are found in parts of the brain that control movement, memory, response to stress, and complex thought—functions that are, not coincidentally, affected by marijuana. Basic research indicates that the body's own cannabinoids play a natural role in all of these processes, as well as in pain perception and the control of nausea and vomiting (see Figure 2.7). Here we will review basic biological evidence that demonstrates how cannabinoids affect movement, memory, pain, nausea, and vomiting. In later chapters we will discuss how these effects have been studied on human patients in clinical settings as they pertain to specific symptoms.

Under the influence of marijuana, many people's bodies sway, and they often have difficulty holding their hands steady. In laboratory experiments, low doses of cannabinoids have been found to stimulate rodents to move around, while larger amounts appeared to inhibit their activity. CB_1 receptors are particularly concentrated in the brain regions that coordinate *movement*, and it is probably these receptors that account for the different effects of

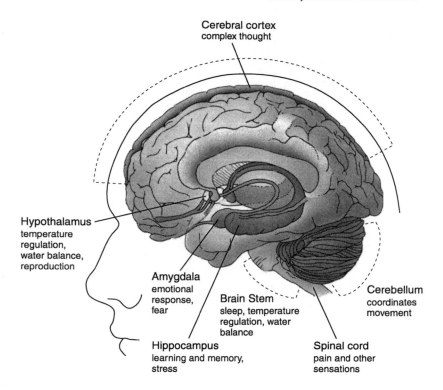

FIGURE 2.7 Locations and functions of brain regions with abundant cannabinoid receptors. Several regions of the brain, which govern a wide range of body functions, contain high concentrations of cannabinoid receptors. Abundant cannabinoid receptors are also present in the following areas not shown in this view of the brain: the basal ganglia, which controls movement; the nucleus of the solitary tract, which governs visceral sensation, nausea, and vomiting; the nucleus acumbens, the brain's reward center; and the central gray area, which registers pain relief.

cannabinoids on movement and activity. The brain regions that coordinate movement include several different sites, among them areas affected by Parkinson's and Huntington's diseases. Because cannabinoids appear to influence movement through a variety of routes, they represent a possible source of new medicines to treat movement disorders.

Marijuana has also been shown to disrupt short-term *memory* in humans. Memory loss probably occurs when cannabinoids flood the abundant CB_1 receptors in the hippocampus, one of the brain's memory centers. In studies of animals and also in experiments on isolated nerve cells, cannabinoids have been found to decrease nerve cell activity and block processes associated with memory formation in the hippocampus. Cannabinoids also appeared to produce temporary effects that resemble injury to that part of the brain. These findings suggest that medicines based on cannabinoids might have undesirable effects on short-term memory due to their action on the hippocampus.

CB_1 receptors are moderately abundant in areas of the brain and spinal cord that control *pain perception*. Animals given cannabinoids in experiments designed to measure their responses to moderate and escapable pain reacted similarly to those given pain-killing opiate drugs, such as morphine. Cannabinoids and opiates have also been shown to provoke comparable chemical responses in nerve cells isolated from the spinal cord; however, the two types of drugs activate different receptors to produce these similar effects. Perhaps because they act at a separate site, cannabinoids—unlike opiates—also appear to block chronic pain sensations in experimental animals. This is an important finding since some types of chronic pain cannot be relieved even by powerful opiate medications.

Cannabinoids also appear to play a role in pain transmission along peripheral nerves, which detect sensations in all parts of the body and relay messages to the brain via the spinal cord. Peripheral nerve cells display both CB_1 and CB_2 receptors on their surfaces, and research in experimental animals indicates that cannabinoids specific to each receptor type appear capable of blocking peripheral nerve pain. These results suggest that a mixture of cannabinoids could enhance each other's effects in relieving peripheral pain in humans. On the other hand, it might be better to design pain relievers that do not bind CB_1 since, as noted above, that receptor type mediates short-term memory loss.

Nausea and vomiting occur under a variety of circumstances, including viral and bacterial infections, emotional distress, and reactions to medications or poisons. Many people claim to have found relief from these symptoms by smoking or ingesting marijuana. Clinical studies indicate that both THC and smoked marijuana can reduce vomiting to some extent, and researchers have found cannabinoid receptors in relative abundance in the part of the brain that controls visceral sensations, including nausea and vomiting. Little is known about how cannabinoids interfere with nausea or vomiting, but their effects clearly differ from those of existing antinausea drugs. Although generally quite effective, conventional medications might theoretically be improved by combining them with cannabinoids. Clinical research will be needed to determine how the different medications would actually interact in patients, however.

CANNABINOIDS AND THE IMMUNE SYSTEM

Through the complex interactions of an elaborate network of organs and cells, the immune system protects the body from bacterial and viral invaders. Because there are so many CB_2 receptors on the different cells that participate in this defense network, cannabinoids are thought to play a role in the immune response (relatively small numbers of CB_1 receptors are also found on immune cells). What role CB_2 might play in immunity, however, remains a mystery—especially since researchers have yet to identify a natural cannabinoid that acts on immune cells much as anandamide acts on nerve cells.

In experiments on animals and isolated cells, cannabinoids have been shown to affect components of the immune system in diverse—and sometimes contradictory—ways. Cannabinoids increase, as well as decrease, certain responses to infection, though it can take up to 10 times more drug to produce these effects than it does to alter nervous system functions. Because most relevant experiments to date have measured the immediate effects of high doses of cannabinoids, the consequences to the immune system of chronic low-level cannabinoid exposure, such as might be found among moderate marijuana users, are unknown.

Nevertheless, basic research on cannabinoids and the immune system has produced several intriguing findings that warrant further study. Many of these reports focus on the effects of THC on one of several species of white blood cells, the workhorses of the immune system. Each type of white blood cell serves a different purpose, and all function in concert to defend the body against disease. Some engulf and destroy foreign substances, some produce antibodies that disable bacteria and viruses, and others issue chemical signals that rally other immune cells to attack and kill invaders.

Several basic studies have provided evidence that cannabinoids can suppress the immune system in a variety of ways, while others have found that cannabinoids can enhance immune responses.[15] Certain natural and synthetic cannabinoids (but not anandamide) have been shown to decrease the ability of some types of white blood cells to multiply in response to infection. Some cannabinoids also appear to depress antibody production under some circumstances and to impede the ability of so-called killer cells to assassinate viruses and bacteria.

In addition to immune suppression caused by cannabinoids, marijuana use poses the additional—and probably greater—risk of immune damage due to smoking. Thus, it is important that future studies on the health risks of medical marijuana use distinguish between adverse effects caused by cannabinoids versus those caused by smoking or other delivery methods.

Chapter 3 discusses these and other potentially harmful effects of marijuana on the immune system. But in some cases the immune system must be suppressed in order to cure disease. Allergies, transplant rejection, and inflammatory disorders all result from immune reactions and thus represent potential targets for cannabinoid therapy. In some experiments, certain cannabinoid drugs have been shown to depress the production of cytokines, hormonelike chemicals that direct immune cells to eliminate foreign substances from the body.

Cannabinoids have also been shown to reduce inflammation and tissue damage in rat brain models of head injury, meningitis, and multiple sclerosis. Relatively little basic research has been conducted in this area, but since many pain medications act by reducing inflammation, this effect could be linked to the apparent ability of cannabinoids to relieve pain.

Following Leads from Basic Research

In recent years researchers have taken important steps toward understanding how chemicals in marijuana affect the cells and tissues of the human body. Many more questions remain to be answered, but the foundation has been laid for even greater advances in the immediate future. In addition to continued basic studies, clinical research on treating pain and movement disorders with cannabinoids appears promising.

The discovery of cannabinoid receptors, and at least some of the compounds that activate these receptors, opens the door to determining what naturally occurring cannabinoids do and how they work. The next logical steps are to pinpoint the location of natural cannabinoids in the brain and to find out how cells produce, store, release, and take them up. This knowledge can lay the groundwork for discovering different cannabinoid drugs with different effects. By following a similar path, medical researchers have learned to harness the benefits and minimize the risks associated with opiate drugs.

Basic studies have also identified several potential health risks associated with marijuana and cannabinoids, which are discussed in the next chapter. These findings, too, should be pursued through ongoing research.

NOTES

1. Abel EL. 1980. *Marihuana: The First Twelve Thousand Years*. New York: Plenum; Aldrich MR. 1997. "History of therapeutic cannabis," in *Cannabis in Medical Practice*, Mathre ML, ed. Jefferson, NC: McFarland; Grinspoon L and Bakalar JB. 1997. *Marihuana: The Forbidden Medicine*. New Haven, CT: Yale University Press.

2. Aldrich MR. 1997.

3. Ibid.; Brunner TF. 1973. "Marijuana in ancient Greece and Rome? The literary evidence." *Bulletin of the History of Medicine* 47:344-355.

4. Rosenthal F. 1971. *The Herb: Hashish Versus Medieval Muslim Society*. Leiden, The Netherlands: Brill.

5. Conrad C. 1993. *Hemp: Lifeline to the Future*. Los Angeles: Creative Xpressions; DuToit BM. 1980. *Cannabis in Africa*. Rotterdam, The Netherlands: Balkema.

6. Aldrich MR. 1997.

7. Abel EL. 1980.

8. Mikuriya TH. 1973. *Marijuana: Medical Papers 1839-1972*. Oakland, CA: Medi-Comp Press.

9. Aldrich MR. 1997; Bonnie RJ and Whitebread CH II. 1974. *The Marihuana Conviction: A History of Marihuana Prohibition in the United States*. Charlottesville: University Press of Virginia.

10. Aldrich MR. 1997.

11. Rosenthal F. 1971.

12. Facklam M and Facklam H. 1992. *Healing Drugs*. New York: Facts on File.

13. Grinspoon L and Bakalar JB. 1997.

14. Taylor HC. 1998. "Analysis of the medical use of marijuana and its social implications." *Journal of the American Pharmaceutical Association* 38(2):220-227.

15. Institute of Medicine. 1999. *Marijuana and Medicine: Assessing the Science Base*. Washington, DC: National Academy Press, p. 60.

HOW HARMFUL IS MARIJUANA?

The most heated arguments over medical marijuana do not concern its ability to alleviate patients' symptoms but rather its potential danger to individual users and to society. This chapter first examines the scientific evidence that marijuana causes physical and psychological injury to individual users. Then it considers the potential social harms that could result from legalizing marijuana for medical uses. More detailed information and complete references for studies described below can be found in Chapter 3 of the 1999 IOM report, *Marijuana and Medicine: Assessing the Science Base.*

WHERE THERE'S SMOKE, THERE'S HARM

Given the well-known consequences of tobacco smoking, it seems logical to suspect that marijuana could be equally detrimental to physical health. Although free of nicotine, marijuana smoke certainly pollutes the lungs. And since tobacco smoking has been linked to respiratory injury, cancer, emphysema, heart disease, complications of pregnancy, low birth weight, and other ills, it makes sense to worry whether smoking marijuana might prove equally harmful.

Scientists have compared marijuana and tobacco smoking on the basis of many different factors but have failed to find consistent evidence that either substance poses a greater health risk than the other. On the one hand, marijuana joints have been shown to deliver at least four times as much tar to the lungs as tobacco cigarettes of equivalent weight. This difference is due to the lack of filters on joints and because marijuana smokers typically inhale a larger volume of smoke and take it more deeply into the lungs than tobacco smokers do. Marijuana smokers also tend to hold smoke in for a time before exhaling, exposing the lungs to even greater levels of cancer-causing agents.

On the other hand, because they are packed more tightly, commercial cigarettes produce more smoke than hand-rolled joints. That, plus the fact that most tobacco users typically smoke more cigarettes per day than their marijuana-using counterparts, means that over the course of a day most tobacco users take far more smoke into their lungs than people who smoke marijuana exclusively. Thus it is impossible to make precise comparisons between the damage to one's health caused by smoking marijuana versus the damage caused by smoking tobacco. And since an estimated 70 percent of marijuana users also smoke tobacco, it is difficult to conduct epidemiological studies that isolate the effects of marijuana smoking.

Not surprisingly, clinical studies suggest that people who smoke marijuana are more likely to develop respiratory illnesses than are nonsmokers. A survey of outpatient medical visits at a large health maintenance organization (HMO) found that marijuana users were more likely to seek help for respiratory illnesses than people who smoked neither marijuana or tobacco.[1] However, the researchers also found that patients who had smoked marijuana for more than 10 years did not seek treatment for respiratory illness with any greater frequency than those who had smoked it for less than 10 years. One possible explanation for this finding is that the people who continued smoking for a long time had not been troubled by respiratory problems such as shortness of breath, while those who did develop uncomfortable symptoms quit smoking relatively quickly. Unfortunately, the marijuana smokers who responded to this survey were not asked if they also used cocaine, which is known to intensify respiratory symptoms. It is also likely that some participants underreported their use of tobacco, alcohol, and marijuana.

A study of 446 volunteers compared the incidence of chronic bronchitis symptoms (excessive cough, sputum production, and wheezing) among habitual marijuana smokers, tobacco smokers, and nonsmokers.[2] Roughly one in three of both the marijuana and the tobacco smokers showed one or more of these symptoms, while only about one in 12 of the nonsmokers did. Smokers—even those who did not smoke tobacco—had episodes of acute bronchitis more than five times as often as nonsmokers. Marijuana smokers also performed worse on lung function tests than did nonsmokers.

The average marijuana smoker in this study consumed three to four joints per day; the tobacco users smoked an average of 20 cigarettes per day. In this study of habitual marijuana smokers, participants who smoked both marijuana and tobacco reported no more symptoms of chronic bronchitis overall than those who smoked tobacco alone, an indication that smoking marijuana does not increase the harms caused by smoking tobacco.

Another study did show evidence of such an interaction, but it was conducted on people who smoked considerably less marijuana and tobacco than those who participated in the previously described study. Researchers have found that, in general, the interactive effects of toxic substances tend to be easiest to detect at low exposure levels. This may explain why the lighter smokers in the second study showed signs of increased respiratory damage when they used both marijuana and tobacco, while the heavier smokers in the first study did not. In any case, both studies indicate that marijuana smoke reduces respiratory function.

Habitual smoking of either marijuana or tobacco damages the lining of the bronchial airways. After continuous exposure to smoke, the delicate tissues along these passageways become red and swollen. Smoking also transforms the cells of the bronchial airways. These passages are normally lined with ciliated cells, whose hairlike projections move rapidly to sweep mucus toward the mouth. But when people smoke, these cells are replaced by others that secrete copious amounts of thick mucus, which can only be expelled by the notorious "smoker's cough."

Bronchial injury, a more sensitive measure of damage than the symptoms of chronic bronchitis, is even greater among people who smoke both marijuana and tobacco. The damage extends to the interiors of bronchial cells, which develop a variety of abnormalities. Some of these changes, which are known to be precursors of cancer, have also been discovered in the respiratory tracts of marijuana and hashish smokers who did not use tobacco.

Another form of respiratory injury caused by tobacco smoke is a condition known as chronic obstructive pulmonary disease (COPD), a slow, progressive loss of elasticity in the passages that deliver air to the lungs. People with COPD become short of breath and exhibit symptoms of chronic bronchitis. Attempts to determine whether marijuana smoke also provokes COPD have produced conflicting results. For example, one group reported that smoking as little as a single joint per day significantly impaired small airway function,[3] while another failed to detect similar damage even in people who smoked four joints a day for more than 10 years.[4] It thus remains to be determined whether chronic marijuana smoking actually causes COPD, but there is good reason to suspect that it does.

While many tobacco smokers accept coughing and shortness of breath as part of the price they pay for the pleasure of smoking, fear of cancer sometimes persuades them to quit. (And then there are people who get little pleasure out of smoking but continue smoking to calm their nerves, that is, to avoid feeling anxious and irritable—the withdrawal symptoms of nicotine addiction.) Whether marijuana users should be similarly concerned remains to be conclusively proven. However, cellular, genetic, and clinical studies all suggest that marijuana smoke is an important risk factor in the development of respiratory cancer.

Many of the same carcinogenic, or cancer-causing, compounds present in tobacco smoke are also found in burning marijuana. In particular, unfiltered smoke from joints contains higher concentrations of a class of chemicals called polycyclic aromatic hydrocarbons (PAHs) than does smoke from tobacco cigarettes. Since marijuana users generally inhale more deeply than tobacco smokers, they may be exposing their lungs to even higher levels of these dangerous substances. Preliminary research also suggests that marijuana smokers' lung cells contain higher levels of an enzyme that converts PAHs into a cancer-causing form. Thus, it is not surprising that several studies implicate marijuana smoking as a risk factor for lung cancer as well as for mouth and throat cancer.

Several reports have suggested that marijuana smokers are at greater risk than nonsmokers of developing cancers in tissues that come into contact with smoke, such as the lungs, mouth, larynx, pharynx, and esophagus. However, these conclusions were based on series of case reports of patients with these cancers rather than from controlled studies. Thus, the increased frequency of cancers among marijuana smokers cannot be attributed to marijuana alone but may also result from other factors, such as tobacco smoking.

To date, only one large-scale study[5] has sought to determine the frequency with which marijuana smokers develop cancer. It included some 65,000 men and women HMO clients between the ages of 15 and 49. Among these people, 1,421 cases of cancer were found, but marijuana use—defined as taking the drug on six or more occasions—appeared to increase only the risk of prostate cancer in men who did not smoke tobacco. No association was found between marijuana use and any other type of cancer, including cancers normally linked to tobacco smoking. However, this study was limited by the fact that many of its participants were younger than the average ages when many cancers appear as well as by the short duration of their marijuana use. Lung cancer, for example, usually develops only after a long exposure to smoking; relatively few marijuana users persist in the habit for more than a few years, and most also smoke tobacco.

Researchers should soon be better able to pursue the question of marijuana's carcinogenicity. More than 30 years have elapsed since the start of widespread marijuana use among young people in the United States, who now constitute a sufficiently large population to support meaningful epidemiological studies. On the other hand, such surveys are difficult to conduct, since far fewer people have smoked marijuana exclusively than have smoked tobacco alone and also because marijuana smokers are likely to underreport their use of the illegal drug.

In contrast to human studies, research on the effects of marijuana smoke at the cellular level provides strong evidence that it contains abundant carcinogens. Exposure to marijuana smoke has been shown to cause chromosomal changes that precede cancer—

and in some cases outright malignancies—in isolated human and animal lung cells. Similar alterations have been detected in the actual lung cells of marijuana smokers and at even higher levels among those who also smoked tobacco.

An especially convincing study evaluated changes in blood cells taken from pregnant women who were exclusive smokers of marijuana and also from their babies after they were born.[6] In a class of white blood cells called lymphocytes, the researchers found significantly more DNA aberrations of a type linked to cancer development as compared with lymphocytes from nonsmoking women and their newborns. In previous studies the same group of investigators had found similar changes in the DNA of tobacco smokers, indicating that the substances responsible for this damage are present in both marijuana smoke and tobacco smoke.

Marijuana smoking has also been associated with increased mortality among men with AIDS. This finding is especially important since such patients comprise the largest group of medical marijuana users in the United States. Several factors may contribute to this trend, which is still largely unexplained. It may be that people who use marijuana also tend to engage in risky sexual behavior or intravenous drug use, either of which puts them at higher risk for developing AIDS, but it is also likely that smoking marijuana adds to the burden that HIV places on the immune system. HIV-seropositive individuals who use marijuana regularly appear to be at increased risk of opportunistic infections and Kaposi's sarcoma; for those who smoke more than one-half pack of cigarettes per day, the risk is somewhat lower. If smoking marijuana indeed makes AIDS patients sicker, it remains to be determined whether smoke, cannabinoids, or both are to blame (see Chapter 5).

THE ROLE OF CANNABINOIDS

The vast majority of studies on the physiological consequences of marijuana use have focused on smoking. However, a few researchers have directly evaluated the effects of cannabinoids on isolated cells, experimental animals, and human subjects. Most such studies have examined one of three areas of potential damage: the immune system, the cardiovascular system, and reproductive and fetal health.

As discussed in the last chapter, several biological studies suggest that cannabinoids can depress the immune system's response to infection. In some experiments, white blood cells in experimental animals exposed to THC and other cannabinoids exhibited a reduced capacity to proliferate following infection; some animals also produced fewer than normal antibodies or showed signs of impaired "killer cell" activity.[7]

Not all studies of this nature implicate cannabinoids as immune suppressants. In fact, some immune functions have been found to increase in response to cannabinoids. Such results are not necessarily contradictory because many physiological processes contribute to immunity. Thus, no single experiment can truly reveal the "big picture" of marijuana's effects on the human immune system. That is particularly true of studies that test the effects of pure cannabinoids such as THC, since marijuana contains a variety of chemicals that may affect immune activity.

Although it demands equally cautious interpretation as studies on individual immune cells, research on disease resistance in animals exposed to cannabinoids more closely tracks the overall impact of cannabinoids on the immune system. Mice infected with pneumonia-causing bacteria died of septic shock when they were injected with THC before and after infection; those that did not receive THC developed immunity to the bacterium and survived. This response was found to vary depending on the amount of THC the mice received and whether it was injected before or after they were infected with the bacteria. Similarly, two doses of THC given before and after infection with the herpes simplex virus appeared to hasten the death of immunodeficient mice, although a single dose of THC prior to infection did not. Both experiments suggest that the timing of THC exposure relative to infection determines whether THC suppresses the immune response.[8]

Even if cannabinoids themselves cause little or no harm to the immune system, there is good reason to believe that smoking marijuana does. Marijuana smoke been linked to increased mortality in people with AIDS and it also appears to injure an important class of immune cells in the lungs. These cells, called alveolar macrophages, are primarily responsible for protecting the lungs against infectious microbes, harmful substances, and tumor cells. Compared with nonsmokers, habitual marijuana smokers in a large study were found to have twice as many alveolar macrophages, a sign that their lungs were fighting infection or invasion. People who smoked both marijuana and tobacco had four times as many of the cells as nonsmokers.[9]

Marijuana smoking was also found to reduce the ability of alveolar macrophages to destroy disease-causing fungus and bacteria as well as tumor cells. Moreover, marijuana smoking appears to depress macrophages' ability to produce cytokines—hormone-like chemicals that help coordinate the immune response.[10] Taken as a whole, these findings indicate that smoking marijuana could have dangerous consequences for patients with compromised immune systems, including people with AIDS and cancer—particularly those who are receiving immunosuppressive chemotherapy—as well as organ transplant recipients.

Exposure to cannabinoids can also affect the cardiovascular system.[11] Although these effects tend to be shortlived, they are far easier to measure than the impact of cannabinoids on the immune system. Both smoked marijuana and THC have been shown to raise heart rate, from 20 to 100 percent above normal in some cases. Oral THC (as well as smoked marijuana) can also exaggerate the drop in blood pressure that occurs when a person rises to standing after lying down, sometimes so much so that the person faints. This reaction rarely occurs after two to three days of repeated exposure to THC or marijuana extract, and it poses little risk for young healthy people. It could, however, present a serious problem for older patients or for people at risk for heart attack or stroke. As chronic marijuana users who began taking the drug during the 1960s approach the age at which cardiovascular disease becomes common, the impact of marijuana use on circulatory health should become clearer. In the meantime, people at risk for cardiovascular disease would be wise to avoid marijuana and THC.

In addition to effects on the immune and cardiovascular systems, researchers have considered the impact of cannabinoids on reproduction.[12] A series of reports involving experimental animals injected with THC indicate that it inhibits several different reproductive functions, from hormone secretion to normal sperm development to embryo implantation. It is important to recognize, however, that most of these studies involved single injections or short-term treatments with the drug, which produced effects that were observed to last for only hours to days. Thus, their results reveal little about the consequences of chronic long-term marijuana or cannabinoid use.

Nevertheless, the few studies that have been conducted to assess THC's effects on human reproduction have produced results that are consistent with those of the animal studies. Fertility research on marijuana users has yielded conflicting results, revealing at worst a short-term depression of reproductive hormones following marijuana use. Over time long-term marijuana users appear to become less sensitive to the inhibitory effects of THC on at least one reproductive factor—luteinizing hormone, which regulates the secretion of testosterone and estrogen. In women the strength of that effect varies with the timing of the menstrual cycle and is most significant between ovulation and the onset of menstruation.

Absent any direct measure of the effects of either marijuana or THC on reproductive function, it seems likely that both substances decrease short-term fertility in men and women. Due to the timing of luteinizing hormone suppression in women, it is also reasonable to predict that THC could interfere with the earliest stages of pregnancy, particularly with embryo implantation. Marijuana smoke appears to pose an even greater threat to pregnant women and couples who are trying to conceive, since it is probably at least as harmful to fetal development as tobacco smoke.

Several epidemiological studies have attempted to trace the effects of marijuana use on pregnancy and fetal development, but their results have been inconsistent. Essentially, the same problems, such as low birth weight, that plague tobacco-smoking mothers and their infants seem to appear among marijuana users. Interestingly, in a study of Jamaican women—who rarely smoke marijuana but prepare it as a tea to relieve morning sickness—no neurobiological or behavioral differences were detected between newborn babies of those who used marijuana and those who did not.[13]

The Ottawa Prenatal Prospective Study has monitored the effects of prenatal marijuana exposure on the cognitive function of children since 1978.[14] So far the study has failed to find evidence that children whose mothers smoked marijuana during pregnancy perform below average on a variety of intelligence tests. Some early cognitive problems were detected among children of women who smoked at least one joint per day during pregnancy, but these deficits were no longer apparent after the children reached age 5. Older children of marijuana users did, however, score slightly lower than those of both nonsmokers and tobacco smokers on tasks that measured their ability to plan ahead and control self-defeating behavior. On the other hand, children whose mothers smoked tobacco during pregnancy scored somewhat lower on tests of language and cognitive skills than the other two groups and continued to do so as late as age 12. In most cases the differences in test scores between groups of comparable children varied by less than 5 percent; thus, the effects, while statistically significant, are subtle.

In summary, there are many reasons to worry that for people who might choose to use marijuana as medicine—and especially those who smoke it—the drug could actually add to their health problems. Proof that habitual marijuana smoking does or does not lead to respiratory cancer awaits the results of extensive, carefully designed epidemiological studies. In the meantime it appears that, for people with chronic medical disorders or those with compromised respiratory or immune systems, smoking marijuana is likely to do more harm than good. Likewise, for people at risk of cardiovascular disease, pregnant women, and couples trying to conceive, the potential risks of either THC or smoked marijuana appear to exceed the potential medical benefits.

Marijuana Abuse

The most talked about health risk associated with marijuana is its potential to promote abuse and addiction. There is great disagreement on this topic and scant evidence that applies specifically to marijuana used solely to relieve medical symptoms. Nevertheless, research from a variety of perspectives—including biological, clinical, and population studies—paints a reasonably detailed picture of the consequences of chronic marijuana use.

Because it is illegal, some people equate any use of marijuana with abuse. The IOM team chose instead to apply the definition of substance abuse used by the medical profession: that people who abuse marijuana use it repeatedly and to their personal detriment. This is the essence of *substance abuse* as described by the *Diagnostic and Statistical Manual of Mental Disorders (DSM-IV)*,[15] the most widely used diagnostic system for mental health care. When people use marijuana compulsively and have trouble stopping despite the fact that their behavior causes severe problems, their diagnosis is more serious than abuse. The DSM-IV classifies such behavior as *substance dependence* (see Box 3.1).

THE PHYSIOLOGY OF USE AND ABUSE

Even marijuana users who do not fit the DSM-IV criteria for abuse or substance dependence may experience symptoms of tolerance, physical dependence, and withdrawal. *Tolerance*, a common response to the repeated use of any drug, occurs when increasing amounts are required to produce a given effect. *Physical dependence* describes the body's adaptation to frequently used drugs. While physical dependence can lead to substance abuse, it does not necessarily do so. If someone who is physically dependent on a drug stops taking it, he or she is likely to experience *withdrawal* symptoms. Most drugs that are abused produce tolerance, physical dependence, and withdrawal—but so do caffeine and nicotine as well as many nonaddictive drugs for pain, anxiety, and high blood pressure. For example, if people who take the medication propranolol for hypertension abruptly stop taking the drug, they are likely to experience withdrawal symptoms that include a temporary rise in blood pressure. To avoid these problems, patients must gradually decrease their dose of propranolol before switching to a different hypertension drug.

Regular marijuana users quickly develop *tolerance* to most of the drug's effects. This may be why heavy users appear to be less impaired than light users after smoking similar amounts of marijuana, despite the finding that heavy users tend to accumulate higher levels of THC in their blood. If users go without marijuana

Box 3.1
DSM-IV Criteria for Substance Dependence

The fourth edition of the *Diagnostic and Statistical Manual of Mental Disorders* (DSM-IV) defines substance dependence as a group of cognitive, behavioral, and physiological symptoms. A person diagnosed with substance dependence meets at least 3 of the following criteria within a twelve-month period:

(1) Tolerance, as defined by either of the following:
   (a) A need for markedly increased amount of the substance to achieve intoxication or desired effect.
   (b) Markedly diminished effect with continued use of the same amount of the substance.
(2) Withdrawal, as defined by either of the following:
   (a) The characteristic withdrawal syndrome for the substance.
   (b) The same (or a closely related) substance is taken to relieve or avoid withdrawal symptoms.
(3) The substance is often taken in larger amounts or over a longer period than was intended.
(4) There is a persistent desire or unsuccessful efforts to cut down or control substance use.
(5) A great deal of time is spent in activities necessary to obtain the substance (e.g., visiting multiple doctors or driving long distances), to use the substance (e.g., chain-smoking), or to recover from its effects.
(6) Important social, occupational, or recreational activities are given up or reduced because of substance use.
(7) The substance use is continued despite knowledge of having a persistent or recurrent physical or psychological problem that is likely to have been caused or exacerbated by the substance (e.g., current cocaine use despite recognition of cocaine-induced depression or continued drinking despite recognition that an ulcer was made worse by alcohol consumption).

Substance abuse with physiological dependence is diagnosed if there is evidence of tolerance or withdrawal.

Substance abuse without physiological dependence is diagnosed if there is no evidence of tolerance or withdrawal.

for a week or so, however, they appear to lose their tolerance to its effects. Interestingly, tolerance to different effects of the same drug can develop at varying rates. Heroin users, for example, become tolerant to the drug's euphoric effects more quickly than they do to its ability to interfere with breathing. Thus, because they tend to increase the amount of drug they take in order to attain the same high, heroin users risk death by asphyxiation.

To our knowledge no marijuana user has ever died of such an overdose. Nevertheless, there are likely to be patients for whom the development of tolerance to cannabinoids would outweigh the benefits of marijuana-based medicines. On the other hand, developing tolerance to certain effects of cannabinoids, such as short-term memory loss or inability to concentrate, could be seen as a benefit. Tolerance to the various cannabinoids may develop at different rates, so it will be important to evaluate their individual effects on mood, movement, memory, and attention if they are to be used as medicines.

People who use marijuana or who take oral THC (e.g., Marinol) appear to become tolerant to some of the drug's effects more quickly than to others. To document this phenomenon, researchers conducted a study of people who smoked marijuana on a daily basis. During the study period, one group of participants smoked marijuana cigarettes four times a day for four consecutive days, while the other group took THC pills on the same schedule. Both thought that the same amount of drug made them feel less and less "high" over the course of four days, but neither group thought that their drug-induced increases in appetite declined over that time. The marijuana-smoking group reported feeling "mellow" after smoking throughout the four days, while the THC-taking group never reported feeling "mellow."[16] The IOM team also heard from several people who had tried both smoked marijuana and oral THC to treat their medical symptoms and whose comparisons of the two drugs resembled those of the study participants.

In addition to human studies, scientists have conducted research on animals to study how tolerance to cannabinoids arises. Like the people in the clinical experiments described above, experimental animals that received THC on an ongoing basis appeared to become tolerant to many of its initial effects, including memory disruption, decreased movement, and pain relief.[17]

Research also indicates that target cells for THC—those that bear CB_1 and CB_2 receptors—adapt to chronic THC exposure in ways that contribute to tolerance. Most studies of brain cells detected a decrease in the production of cannabinoid receptors under conditions that mimicked prolonged exposure to cannabinoids. Tolerance to cannabinoids appears to develop at different rates in different regions of the brain, however, which may explain why a few such studies have *not* found a decline in cannabinoid receptors. This phenomenon could also explain why tolerance to some effects of THC develops more quickly than to other effects. And in addition to their effects on CB_1 and CB_2 receptors, cannabinoids may have a desensitizing effect on other proteins in target cells.

Although intriguing, the results of these and other basic studies on the effects of cannabinoids should be interpreted with caution. Most basic studies consist of short-term experiments that merely simulate long-term marijuana use by exposing animals to higher amounts of cannabinoids than typically experienced by marijuana users. Moreover, cannabinoids behave differently in the human body depending on whether they are inhaled, injected, or swallowed. While most people ingest cannabinoids by smoking, they are generally injected into laboratory animals. Still, some of the same biochemical responses to chronic cannabinoid exposure that have been observed in experimental animals probably occur in humans as well, though perhaps in subtler forms.

Withdrawal from either marijuana or THC has been shown to cause several distinct symptoms, as reported by participants in clinical studies and adolescents undergoing treatment for substance abuse. These include restlessness, irritability, mild agitation, insomnia, sleep disturbance, nausea, and cramping—uncomfortable sensations, to be sure, but far milder than symptoms associated with alcohol withdrawal (see Table 3.1). Following very high doses of oral THC—the equivalent of smoking between five and 10 joints of average potency per day for 10 to 20 days— withdrawal symptoms also included runny nose, sweating, and decreased appetite, but lasted only four days.[18] In another study,

TABLE 3.1 Common Withdrawal Symptoms Produced by Various Drugs

	Marijuana	Nicotine	Alcohol	Cocaine	Opiates (morphine and heroin)
Irritability	X	X	X		X
Low Mood, Depression		X		X	X
Anxiety		X			X
Sleep Disturbance	X	X	X	X	X
Nausea	X		X		X
Cramps	X				X
Increased or Decreased Heart Rate		X	X	X	
Craving		X	X	X	X

Source: O'Brien CP. 1996. Drug addiction and drug abuse. In: Harmon JG, Limbird LE, Molinoff PB, Ruddon RW, Gilman AG, Editors *Goodman and Gilman's The Pharmacological Basis of Therapeutics.* 9th Edition. New York: McGraw-Hill. Pp. 557-577.

participants took about half as much THC for only four days but reported that their withdrawal symptoms lasted longer.[19]

In animals, simply administering THC for several days or weeks and then discontinuing it does not provoke withdrawal symptoms because the drug lingers in the brain, allowing it to gradually adapt. A similar situation probably occurs in human marijuana users who go "cold turkey," easing the process of withdrawal. However, by administering a chemical block that immediately interferes with THC's effects, researchers can create a sort of instantaneous withdrawal in experimental animals that have been chronically exposed to THC. These animals exhibit dramatic symptoms, including hyperactivity and disorganized behavior, which also occur during withdrawal from opiate drugs.

Tolerance and withdrawal certainly contribute to a drug's capacity for abuse. But ultimately the better a drug makes people feel, the more likely they are to abuse it. This effect, called *reinforcement*, generally depends on drug dosage. Caffeine, for example, is reinforcing for many people who drink a cup or two of coffee at a time but is *aversive*—that is, it makes most people feel worse, not better—if they consume the caffeine equivalent of six cups of coffee all at once. Reinforcement for a particular drug also varies from person to person. In the case of caffeine, research indicates that its effects are the most pleasurable for the least anxious people.

Marijuana is indisputably reinforcing to many people. Some have argued that marijuana has a relatively low potential for abuse, based on experiments in which animals—who willingly dose themselves with cocaine—did not self-administer THC. Other studies indicate that THC *is* rewarding to animals in relatively mild doses but that, like many reinforcing drugs, it is aversive in large amounts. Cannabinoids have also been shown to unleash a surge of dopamine, a chemical generally associated with reinforcement, in rats; however, the mechanism by which cannabinoids exert this effect appears to be different from that of other abused drugs such as cocaine and heroin. It is also important to note that the dopamine "reward" system in the brain responds to a wide variety of stimuli, not all of which are dangerous substances. For example, from animal studies we know that dopamine levels also rise in response to feelings of sexual attraction and when eating sweet foods. Based on similarities in brain structure and function, this is probably true of humans as well.

As people progress from tolerance to physical dependence to drug abuse, their *craving* intensifies despite mounting problems caused by their behavior. This intense desire for a drug is the toughest part of addiction to overcome. As a result, most recovering addicts suffer a relapse within one year of becoming drug-free. Animal studies suggest that this tendency to relapse results from long-term changes in brain function brought on by addiction. These alterations appear to persist for months or years after the last use of an addictive drug.

Anticraving medications have been developed for nicotine and alcohol, while methadone reduces cravings for heroin as it blocks the drug's euphoric effects.

Research on cravings has focused on nicotine, alcohol, cocaine, and opiate drugs. It has not specifically addressed marijuana, so it remains unknown whether marijuana induces similar changes in brain function.

MARIJUANA USE AND DEPENDENCE

Another way to look at the risk of marijuana addiction is to examine general patterns of use and dependence. Who uses marijuana? How frequently and under what circumstances do marijuana users become abusers? How do patterns of marijuana abuse compare with those of other abused substances? Social scientists and epidemiologists have addressed several aspects of these questions in recent years.

Millions of Americans have tried marijuana, but most do not use it regularly. According to a U.S. Department of Health and Human Services household survey conducted in 1997, 33 percent of the U.S. population over the age of 12 (some 70 million people) has tried marijuana or hashish at least once. Only 5 percent of respondents reported that they currently use either substance. Marijuana use was most prevalent among people between 18 and 25 and declined sharply in people age 34 and older.

These results fit a long-observed scenario: many people try marijuana as adolescents, but few continue to use it past young adulthood (see Figure 3.1). Peer pressure, as well as the desire to conform or appear mature, typically prompts teenagers to try marijuana for the first time. Different factors, however, appear to influence marijuana use beyond mere experimentation.

In one study of 456 students who tried marijuana while in high school, those who became regular (but not heavy) marijuana users typically said they continued to take the drug to improve their mood, rather than for any social reason.[20] This finding is in keeping with additional research on young adults, who tend to use drugs on a regular basis to satisfy psychological needs rather than to impress others.

Only 28 percent of the high school students continued using marijuana after their initial experimentation with the drug. Several who quit did so because they felt that marijuana had harmed either their health or their relationships with other people. Some

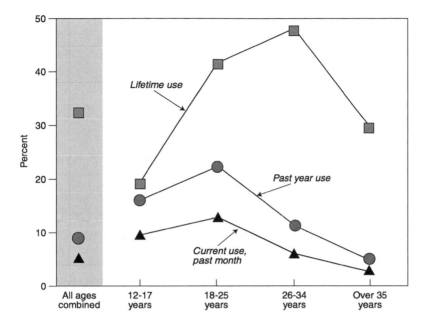

FIGURE 3.1 Age distribution of marijuana users among the general population in 1996. (Adapted from *Marijuana and Medicine: Assessing the Science Base*. Institute of Medicine. 1999. Washington, DC: National Academy Press.)

said they stopped when they found themselves in positions of responsibility or in less frequent contact with other marijuana users. They also cited parental disapproval more often than peer disapproval as a factor in their decision to give up marijuana.

But people who turn to marijuana to relieve medical symptoms—most of whom are older than 35—face an entirely different set of circumstances than do youthful recreational users. There are no existing scientific studies of the relationship between medical marijuana use and abuse. However, several individual and environmental factors appear to influence whether a particular person is likely to abuse or become addicted to a given drug. Each of these criteria bears consideration in calculating the risks posed by medical marijuana.

Some segments of the population appear to be more susceptible to drug dependence in general than others. For example, national survey results indicate that men are 1.6 times more likely to become dependent on illicit drugs than are women. The risk of drug dependence for white Americans is approximately double that for African Americans. People between the ages of 25 and 44 are estimated to be more than three times as likely than those over 45 to abuse drugs.

Adolescents are particularly vulnerable to drug dependence since they tend to suffer the behavioral consequences of dependence at lower levels of drug use compared with adults. Young people who are already dependent on other substances—typically alcohol or tobacco—are especially prone to marijuana dependence. In a study of more than 200 patients in a residential treatment program for delinquent youth, participants were found to be dependent on an average of more than three different substances. Of those patients who had used marijuana more than six times, more than 80 percent went on to become dependent on it—a far higher rate of progression to dependence than found among the general population.[21]

Although parents of children who use marijuana often claim that the drug provokes rebellious behavior, the adolescents in the previous study had all displayed behavioral problems *before* they began abusing marijuana. Several other reports echo these observations and indicate that the more troubled a child is, the earlier he or she is likely to begin drug use, abuse, and dependence.

People with psychiatric disorders constitute another group at high risk for drug abuse. An estimated 76 percent of men and 65 percent of women classified as being drug dependent suffer from at least one additional psychiatric disorder; most frequently, that disorder is alcohol abuse. In drug-dependent women, phobias and major depression are nearly as common as alcohol abuse. Antisocial personality and its predecessor in children, conduct disorder, also figure prominently in the psychiatric diagnoses of substance abusers.

Genetic factors also appear to influence whether a person will abuse drugs, including marijuana. A study of over 8,000 male twins indicates that people inherit the tendency to enjoy marijuana's effects.[22] Presumably, people who try marijuana and find it pleasant are more likely to continue using it—and thus possibly abuse it—than those who do not find it enjoyable. The results of this study and a similar survey of female twins[23] indicate that some people who experiment with marijuana may be genetically predisposed to becoming regular users. Whether a person ever tries marijuana, however, appears to be most strongly influenced by one's family and social environment.

Although marijuana seems to pose an increased risk of abuse for some people, it is generally considered to be only mildly addictive. Compared with users of several other addicting substances, few people who use marijuana become dependent on it (see Figure 3.2). Thus, while many more people try—and use—marijuana than other illicit drugs such as cocaine or heroin, marijuana abuse cases are relatively rare. Two large-scale surveys—the National Comorbidity Survey[24] and the Epidemiological Catchment Area Program[25]—have found that about 5 percent of the U.S. population has been dependent on marijuana at some

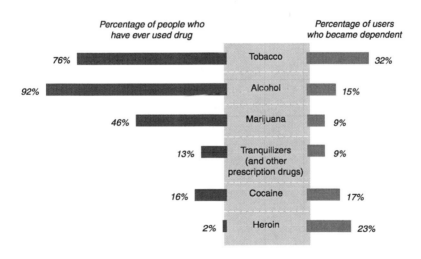

FIGURE 3.2 Prevalence of drug use and dependence in the general population. The higher estimates for marijuana use shown here compared to those reported by the Department of Health and Human Services household survey shown in Figure 3.1 are probably due to differences in how the surveys were conducted. (Adapted from J.C. Anthony, L.A. Warner, R.C. Kessler. 1994. Comparative epidemiology of dependence on tobacco, alcohol, controlled substances, and inhalants: Basic findings from the National Comorbidity Survey. *Experimental and Clinical Psychopharmacology* 2:244-268.)

point in their lives. By comparison, nearly 14 percent of adults met the criteria for dependence on alcohol and 36 percent met the criteria for tobacco dependence.

Clearly, marijuana use carries a risk of dependence and abuse—a danger that must be taken into account if either the crude plant extract or its active ingredients are to be used for medical purposes. For certain patients—particularly adolescents, people with psychological or social problems, and those with an inherited predisposition to substance abuse—marijuana-based medications may not be worth the risk. On the other hand, compared with alcohol, tobacco, and several prescription medications, marijuana's abuse potential appears relatively small and certainly within manageable limits for patients under the care of a physician.

PSYCHOLOGICAL HARMS

Compared with the physical dangers of marijuana use, its psychological drawbacks are far less well understood. Indeed, some of the psychoactive effects of marijuana—such as anxiety reduction, sedation, and euphoria—can be counted among the drug's potential benefits for certain patients. This paradox, plus the fact that the vast majority of research on the psychological effects of marijuana and cannabinoids concerns intoxication and recreational use, makes it difficult to anticipate the psychological impact of medical marijuana use.

One would expect that people who use marijuana solely as a medicine have very different mental experiences than those of recreational users simply because the circumstances under which people use psychoactive drugs strongly influence their psychological reactions. Most of the existing psychological research on marijuana was conducted on people who had previously used the drug, so very little is known about its potential to cause adverse psychological reactions in first-time or inexperienced users. Moreover, the majority of psychological studies have measured the effects of a single, often large, dose of the drug, rather than the chronic exposure that would be more typical of medical use. Instead, it is the subtler effects of low doses of marijuana and cannabinoids that must be taken into account if they are to be used as the basis for medications. For even in amounts too small to cause users to feel "high," marijuana and THC provoke changes in mood, thinking, and performance on tasks that demand a combination of attention and coordination.

Marijuana's popularity as a recreational drug hinges on its ability to induce a temporary sense of well-being or euphoria in most users. Many feel that being high enhances their physical and emotional sensitivity, causing them to become talkative and more engaged with other people. Because it suppresses short-term memory and learning, though, people under the influence of marijuana often have difficulty carrying on an intelligible conversation. Short-term memory loss also causes distortions in their sense of time.

Adverse mood reactions to marijuana also can occur, particularly among inexperienced users after smoking or eating a large dose. The most common among such acute reactions are anxiety and paranoia; others include panic, depression, depersonalization, delusions, illusions, and hallucinations. These symptoms usually disappear within hours and respond well to reassurance and a supportive environment. Seventeen percent of regular marijuana smokers report that they have experienced at least one of these symptoms at some time—typically early in their use of the drug.[26]

Large doses of marijuana also impair cognition. Using an imaging technique called positron emission tomography to measure the acute effects of marijuana on brain function, researchers have detected blood-flow abnormalities in volunteers after they smoked a single marijuana cigarette; specifically, circulation to the temporal lobe of the brain, which governs auditory attention, was restricted. This effect coincided with diminished performance in listening tasks. Yet smoking marijuana also appears to increase, not decrease, blood flow to the brain's frontal lobes and lateral cerebellum. The frontal lobes control a variety of cognitive functions, including abstract thinking, and are also involved in motor control and emotional reactions; the cerebellum coordinates movement and also governs some types of learning.[27] The science of measuring activity in the living brain is still new. It is not entirely clear what these intriguing changes in cerebral blood flow indicate, but they seem to support the general contention that marijuana impairs thinking.

In the 1970s, reports suggested that heavy marijuana use causes structural changes in the brain, but this finding has not been confirmed when examined with more sophisticated techniques. While more recent studies have found that heavy marijuana users make subtle mistakes in cognitive tasks after they abstain from the drug for 19 to 24 hours, some researchers have questioned the validity of this conclusion because the users may not have been matched against nonusers with comparable cognitive abilities.[28]

Marijuana has also been shown to affect activities that require a fine balance of attention and muscular coordination, such as driving. Such functions are governed by psychomotor processes, which include the ability to control body and limb movement, sustain attention, and respond to environmental cues with appropriate movements. A study of experienced airplane pilots showed that their performance on flight simulator tests was impaired as long as 24 hours after smoking a single marijuana cigarette. Interestingly, prior to taking the test the pilots told investigators that they were sure their performance would not be affected.[29]

Clearly, the evidence that marijuana impairs cognitive and psychomotor performance indicates that medical users will need to limit their activities—much as after taking a strong painkiller or drinking alcohol. No one under the influence of marijuana or THC should drive a vehicle or operate potentially dangerous equipment.

One of the most controversial effects that marijuana has been claimed to produce is a so-called amotivational syndrome. Although this syndrome is not a medical diagnosis, it has been used to describe the behavior of young people who lose interest in school, work, and social activities. When heavy marijuana use accompanies this behavior, the drug is often cited as the cause, despite the fact that no convincing data demonstrate that marijuana actually provokes these symptoms.

It is not enough to observe that chronic marijuana users lack drive or ambition. In order to justify such a claim, people's behavior and personality traits must be compared before and after they become regular users. Because it would be unethical to encourage a person to use marijuana heavily, such research can only be conducted on people who become users on their own. An epidemiological survey could be used to identify such young people and might shed light on the relationship between motivation and marijuana use. But while such a study might show that marijuana users tend to lose motivation compared with nonusers, it could not be used to establish that marijuana use *causes* people to become unmotivated.

A major question remains as to whether marijuana can produce severe and lasting psychotic disorders. There are clinical reports of marijuana-induced states that resemble psychoses such as schizophrenia, depression, and mania, with symptoms that last a week or more. Some researchers have argued that the diversity of these symptoms belies the existence of a specific "marijuana psychosis." Others have concluded that heavy marijuana use—and perhaps even acute use in especially sensitive people—can produce a psychosis characterized by a suite of symptoms such as confusion, amnesia, delusions, hallucinations, anxiety, and agitation. Regardless of which of these interpretations is correct, both camps agree that marijuana use alone—without the influence of additional risk factors—is unlikely to provoke a psychosis that persists longer than intoxication.[30]

Drug abuse is common among people with mental illness. Thus, it is not surprising that several (but not all) studies have shown that a disproportionately large number of people with schizophrenia use marijuana. The association between marijuana and schizophrenia is not well understood, however. While experts generally agree that heavy marijuana use can provoke schizophrenic episodes in susceptible individuals, they also concur that the drug does not cause the underlying disorder. Additional research indicates that people with schizophrenia prefer the effects of marijuana over those produced by alcohol and cocaine, which they generally use less often than does the general population. The reasons for this preference remain unknown, but it suggests that marijuana might give these patients some relief from their symptoms. But people with schizophrenia or a family history of the disease should understand that using marijuana puts them at a greater than average risk for adverse psychiatric reactions.[31]

Some of marijuana's psychological effects may prove to be

medically useful. For example, the antianxiety properties of cannabinoids may help relieve conditions worsened by anxiety, such as movement disorders or nausea. It is also possible that the euphoric good feelings of the marijuana high could enhance the benefits of marijuana-based medicines for pain relief or appetite stimulation. On the other hand, cannabinoid-induced euphoria or sedation may simply mask symptoms, leading some users to the false belief that marijuana improves their medical conditions. That is a problem if it causes patients to choose marijuana over more effective conventional medicines that have fewer undesirable side effects. Thus, the IOM researchers recommended that any future clinical trials of cannabinoid drugs include an evaluation of their psychological impact.

MEDICAL MARIJUANA: A DANGER TO SOCIETY?

Almost everyone who spoke or wrote to the IOM study team about medical marijuana's potential harms felt that acknowledgment of marijuana's possible medical value would undermine its reputation as a dangerous drug, particularly among young people. Yet if marijuana-based drugs were to be developed, they would join a wide variety of effective medications known to be dangerous if misused. While it is important to explore the various ways that medical use of marijuana might encourage drug abuse, it must also be recognized that marijuana is hardly unique among medicines in carrying a burden of risk.

The question is not so much whether marijuana can be both harmful and helpful but whether public perception of its benefits will lead to increased abuse. There is also the concern that experience with marijuana may prompt people to use harder drugs, triggering a general rise in the abuse of illegal substances.

Those who depict marijuana as a so-called gateway drug recognize that other illicit drugs, such as cocaine or heroin, are even more dangerous to both individual health and society as a whole. The gateway concept also reflects strikingly consistent patterns of drug use from adolescence to adulthood. Because it is the most widely used illegal drug, marijuana is predictably the first one that most people encounter, including users who later turn to other illicit substances. Before experimenting with marijuana, however, most future drug users become well acquainted with alcohol and nicotine—usually when they are too young to do so legally.

Discussions of marijuana as a gateway drug usually refer to—and often confuse—two distinct behavioral scenarios. The first, more often called the "stepping stone" hypothesis, is the notion that marijuana possesses pharmacological properties that compel users to experiment with harder drugs. The second and more common theory is that marijuana opens a door to the world of illegal substances. Once introduced to illicit drug use via marijuana, young people encounter increased peer pressure to try other drugs and gain easier access to them.

The stepping-stone hypothesis applies to marijuana only in the sense that individuals who enjoy marijuana's effects probably have a stronger than average attraction to mood-altering substances. In other words, many of the same factors that induce people to use marijuana are likely to predispose them to use harder drugs as well. Those factors include physiological reactions to drugs, the psychological state of the user, and the social context in which the drug is used. Additional factors are addressed by the gateway theory, which asserts that marijuana, due to its illegal status, serves as a conduit to harder drugs.

People who are most likely to use illicit drugs other than marijuana tend to share several traits, including use of alcohol or nicotine at an early age, heavy marijuana use, and psychiatric disorders. Yet while it appears that people who try alcohol and nicotine earliest are more likely than others to experiment with illegal drugs, they are no more likely to become heavy drug users. Similarly, experimental or infrequent users of marijuana are less likely to progress to harder drug use than those who smoke marijuana on a daily basis. One study of young adult males found that those who had used marijuana between 10 and 99 times in their lives were unlikely to have tried another illicit drug, while more than half of those who had used marijuana more than 100 times had done so.[32]

Data that have been collected on the gateway phenomenon are frequently overinterpreted. For example, in one study, researchers concluded that "marijuana's role as a gateway drug appears to have increased" based on interviews with drug abusers who reported using crack cocaine or heroin daily.[33] However, only a tiny fraction of the adult population—an estimated one to three per 1,000 people—uses crack or heroin this often. While most of the people interviewed for the study said they had used marijuana before moving on to harder drugs, that trend is not necessarily true among marijuana users in general.

Another drawback of many studies on the gateway theory is that they rely on measurements of drug use rather than drug dependence. Thus, these studies can only demonstrate that, when compared with people who have never used the drug, marijuana users are more likely to try other drugs as well; such studies do not prove that marijuana users tend to become dependent, or even frequent, users of harder drugs. The real value of this type of research is that it can reveal factors that predict whether a person will progress from using a given illegal drug to a harder one.

Marijuana is a gateway drug in the sense that its use typically precedes rather than follows initiation into other illicit substances. On the other hand, marijuana use per se does not appear to be a gateway to the extent that it is a cause, or even a significant predictor, of hard drug abuse. Instead, the most consistent predictors of hard drug abuse appear to be *intense* marijuana use, psychiatric disorders, and a family history of psychological problems or alcoholism.

It is also important to recognize that research on drug progression has focused exclusively on recreational use. It does not follow that if marijuana were available by prescription for medical use the pattern of subsequent drug progression among medical users would be the same as for recreational users. In fact, a study of nonmedical use of psychoactive prescription drugs—including tranquilizers, antidepressants, and opiate painkillers—failed to find that a clear or consistent sequence of drug use following the abuse of these medications. At present, data on drug use neither support nor refute the assertion that legalizing marijuana for medical purposes would prompt increased drug abuse among medical marijuana users.

A related but distinct concern is whether the use of marijuana for medical purposes would encourage drug use throughout society in general. Unless and until marijuana is approved for medical treatment, we can only speculate about the answer to this question. However, reasonable inferences can be drawn about the outcome of such a change based on three examples: patterns of abuse for opiate drugs, including painkillers such as morphine and codeine; patterns of drug abuse in the Netherlands and also in some parts of the United States, where marijuana was decriminalized in the 1970s; and the short-term consequences of the campaign to legalize medical marijuana in California in 1996.

Opiates can be considered a "stand-in" for marijuana-based medicines since both classes of drugs have the potential to be abused to great harm as well as to be used for medical benefit. Earlier in this century some physicians raised concerns that liberal use of opiates would cause many patients to become addicted to the drugs. Such worries have proven unfounded, and it is now widely recognized that physicians often needlessly limit doses of opiate medications to patients in pain out of fear of producing addicts. Today, opiates are carefully regulated by medical caregivers and rarely diverted from legitimate use to the black market.

There is no evidence to suggest that the use of opiates or cocaine for medical purposes has increased the perception that the illicit use of these drugs is safe or acceptable. Clearly, some patients may abuse these substances for their psychoactive effects, and others may divert them to recreational users. The same problems have occurred with several other medications, most of which are included in Schedule II of the Controlled Substances Act. Both the dispensation and manufacturing of Schedule II drugs are strictly controlled, and physicians are cautioned to monitor their use by patients who may be at risk for drug abuse.

Two studies designed to probe the effects of marijuana decriminalization have reported somewhat conflicting conclusions. Monitoring the Future, an annual survey of high school seniors, revealed that students in states that had decriminalized marijuana did not report using the drug more than their counterparts in states where marijuana remained illegal between 1975 and 1980.[34] Another study, based on drug-related emergency room (ER) cases, concluded that decriminalization had increased marijuana use.[35] It indicated that among states that had decriminalized marijuana in 1975-1976, there was a greater increase between 1975 and 1978 in the number of ER patients who had used marijuana than in states that did not decriminalize the drug.

However, the study also found that by 1978 the *proportion* of marijuana users among ER patients was about equal in states that did and did not decriminalize marijuana; prior to decriminalization, states in which marijuana continued to remain illegal had higher rates of marijuana use than those that eventually legalized the drug. In contrast to marijuana use, rates of other illicit drug use among ER patients were substantially higher in states that did not decriminalize marijuana. Thus, there is more than one possible explanation for the relatively greater increase in marijuana use in the decriminalized states: on the one hand, decriminalization may have led to an increased use of marijuana; on the other hand, where marijuana remained illegal, people may have been less likely to discriminate between it and other illicit substances, a view that would tend to increase the use of hard drugs.

In 1976 the Netherlands adopted a policy making it legal for individuals to possess up to 30 grams of marijuana. Research indicates that little change in marijuana use occurred for seven years following this change in policy; however, in 1984, when "coffee shops" that sold marijuana began to spread throughout Amsterdam, marijuana use started to increase. During the 1990s, marijuana use continued to increase in the Netherlands at the same rate as in the United States and Norway—two countries that strictly forbid the sale and possession of marijuana. Nearly equal percentages of American and Dutch 18 year olds were found to have used marijuana during this period, while Norwegian 18 year olds were about half as likely to have used marijuana. Although these results offer little evidence that the Dutch decriminalization policy itself led to increased levels of marijuana use, it appears that the commercialization of marijuana sales may have done so.

According to the most recent National Household Survey on Drug Abuse, significantly fewer children between the ages of 12 and 17 reported that they perceived marijuana as a "great risk of harm" in 1997 than in 1996.[36] At first glance this might seem to validate the fear that the medical marijuana debate of 1996—prior to passage of the California medical marijuana referendum in November 1997—had caused more teenagers to believe that marijuana use is safe. But a closer analysis of the data show that, despite exposure to a statewide advertising campaign in favor of medical marijuana, teens in California were actually an exception to the national trend: their perception of marijuana's harmfulness did not decrease between 1996 and 1997. Thus, there is no evidence that the medical marijuana debate has altered adolescents' perceptions of the risks of using marijuana.[37]

WEIGHING MARIJUANA'S HARMS

For most people the main adverse effect of *acute* marijuana use—that is, the immediate effect of a single potent dose—is diminished psychomotor performance. A few people also experience bad feelings that range from uneasiness to profound emotional discomfort. Marijuana and marijuana-based drugs pose a greater danger to people at risk for psychiatric disorders, especially those who are vulnerable to substance dependence. This spectrum of risk for acute side effects lies well within tolerable limits for prescription medications.

An even more important concern about medical marijuana is the drug's *chronic* side effects (those that crop up during extended use). These effects fall into two categories: the long-term consequences of smoking and the risks of chronic exposure to THC. Marijuana smoke, like tobacco smoke, is associated with increased risk of cancer, lung damage, and poor pregnancy outcomes. Smoked marijuana is thus unlikely to prove to be a safe medication for any chronic medical condition.

A less prevalent side effect of protracted marijuana use is dependence, which tends to occur only in a vulnerable subpopulation of users, most notably adolescents with conduct disorder. As one might expect, people with psychiatric problems and those vulnerable to substance abuse may be at risk of becoming dependent on medical marijuana.

In addition to the dangers of smoke inhalation, another drawback of using marijuana cigarettes as a drug delivery system is their highly variable composition. Plants grown under different conditions contain variable mixtures of cannabinoids, and their dried leaves may also be contaminated with toxic bacteria and fungus.

As for the notion that the sanctioning of medical marijuana

might lead to an increase in its nonmedical use or to drug abuse in general, no convincing data exist that support this concern. Research suggests that, if marijuana were as closely regulated as other medications with abuse potential, it would pose no special threat of increased abuse; however, no existing study has directly addressed this question. Even if it could be demonstrated that medical use of marijuana would decrease the perception that it can cause harm, this evidence would not be pertinent to the legal regulation of marijuana-based therapeutics. Whether a drug gains federal approval for medical use hinges on its safety and efficacy for individual use, not the perceptions or beliefs it engenders in society at large.

Marijuana is not, to be sure, a completely benign substance. It is a powerful drug that affects the body and mind in a variety of ways. However, except for the damage caused by smoking marijuana, its adverse effects resemble those of many approved medications. While the effectiveness of marijuana-based medicines remains largely to be determined, existing clinical data suggest that marijuana and its component chemicals could contribute to the treatment of numerous disorders. Part II of this book explores the potential of marijuana and cannabinoids to relieve the symptoms of several specific conditions.

NOTES

1. Polen MR, Sidney S, Tekawa IS, Sadler M, Friedman D. 1993. "Health care use by frequent marijuana smokers who do not smoke tobacco." *The Western Journal of Medicine* 158:596-601.

2. Tashkin DP, Coulson AH, Clark VA, Simmons M, Bourque LB, Duann S, Spivey GH, Gong H. 1987. "Respiratory symptoms and lung function in habitual, heavy smokers of marijuana alone, smokers of marijuana and tobacco, smokers of tobacco alone, and nonsmokers." *American Review of Respiratory Disease* 135:205-216.

3. Ammenheuser MM, Berenson AB, Babiak AE, Singleton CR, Whorton EB Jr. 1998. "Frequencies of *hprt* mutant lymphocytes in marijuana-smoking mothers and their newborns." *Mutation Research* 403:55-64.

4. Tashkin DP, et al. 1987.

5. Sidney S, Quesenberry CP Jr, Friedman GD, Tekawa IS. 1997. "Marijuana use and cancer incidence (California, United States)." *Cancer Cause and Control* 8:722-728.

6. Ammenheuser MM, et al. 1998.

7. Institute of Medicine. 1999. *Marijuana and Medicine: Assessing the Science Base.* Washington, DC: National Academy Press, pp. 59-68.

8. Ibid.

9. Barbers RG, Gong HJ, Tashkin DP, Oishsi J, Wallace JM. 1987. "Differential examination of bronchoalveolar lavage cells in tobacco cigarette and marijuana smokers." *American Review of Respiratory Disease* 135:1271-1275.

10. Institute of Medicine. *Marijuana and Medicine.* pp. 112-113.

11. Ibid., pp. 121-122.

12. Ibid., pp. 122-125.

13. Dreher MC, Nugent K, Hudgins R. 1994. "Prenatal marijuana exposure and neonatal outcomes in Jamaica: An ethnographic study." *Pediatrics* 93:254-260.

14. Fried, PA. 1995. "The Ottawa Prenatal Prospective Study (OPPS): Methodological issues and findings." *Life Sciences* 56:2159-2168.

15. American Psychiatric Association. 1994. *Diagnostic and Statistical Manual of Mental Disorders (DSM-IV).* Fourth edition. Washington, DC: American Psychiatric Association.

16. Haney M, Ward AS, Comer SD, Foltin RW, Fischman MW. 1999. "Abstinence symptoms following oral THC administration in humans." *Psychopharmacology* 141:385-404.

17. Childers SR, Breivogel CS. 1998. "Cannabis and endogenous cannabinoid systems." *Drug and Alcohol Dependence* 51:173-187.

18. Jones, RT, Benowitz N, Bachman J. 1976. "Clinical studies of tolerance and dependence." *Annals of the New York Academy of Sciences* 282:221-239.

19. Dreher MC, et al. 1994.

20. Bailey SL, Flewelling RL, Rachal JV. 1992. "Predicting continued use of marijuana among adolescents: The relative influence of drug-specific and social context factors." *Journal of Health and Social Behavior* 33:51-66.

21. Crowley TJ, Macdonald MJ, Whitmore EA, Mikulich SK. 1998. "Cannabis dependence, withdrawal, and reinforcing effects among adolescents with conduct symptoms and substance use disorders." *Drug and Alcohol Dependence* 50:27-37.

22. Lyons MJ, Toomey R, Meyer JM, Green AI, Eisen SA, Goldberg J, True WR, Tsuang MT. 1997. "How do genes influence marijuana use? The role of subjective effects." *Addiction* 92:409-417.

23. Kendler SA and Prescott CA. 1998. "Cannabis use, abuse, and dependence in a population-based sample of female twins." *American Journal of Psychiatry* 155:1016.

24. Anthony JD, Warner LA, Kessler RC. 1994. "Comparative epidemiology of dependence on tobacco, alcohol, controlled substances and inhalants: Basic findings from the National Comorbidity Survey." *Experimental and Clinical Psychopharmacology* 2:244-268.

25. Robins LN and Regier DA, eds. 1991. *Psychiatric Disorders in America: The Epidemiologic Catchment Area Study.* New York: Free Press.

26. Institute of Medicine. *Marijuana and Medicine*, p. 84.

27. Ibid., p. 106.

28. Ibid., pp. 106-107.

29. Yeasavage JA, Leirer VO, Denari M, Hollister LE. 1985. "Carry-over effects of marijuana intoxication on aircraft pilot performance: A preliminary report." *American Journal of Psychiatry* 142:1325-1329.

30. Institute of Medicine. *Marijuana and Medicine*, pp. 105-106.

31. Yeasavage JA, et al. 1985.

32. Institute of Medicine. *Marijuana and Medicine*, p. 100.

33. Golub A and Johnson BD. 1994. "The shifting importance of alcohol and marijuana as gateway substances among serious drug abusers." *Journal of Studies on Alcohol* 55:607-614.

34. Johnston LD, O'Malley PM, Bachman JG. 1989. "Marijuana decriminalization: The impact on youth, 1975-1980." *Journal of Public Health* 10:456.

35. Model KE. 1993. "The effect of marijuana decriminalization on hospital emergency room drug episodes: 1975-1978." *Journal of the American Statistical Association* 88:737-747.

36. Substance Abuse and Mental Health Services Administration. 1998. *National Household Survey on Drug Abuse: Population Estimates 1997.* DHHS Pub. No. (SMA) 98-3250. Rockville, MD: SAMHSA, Office of Applied Studies.

37. Institute of Medicine. *Marijuana and Medicine*, p. 104.

II

MEDICAL MARIJUANA AND DISEASE

W hile most conventional medications reach the public only after an extensive process of development and testing (see Chapter 10), medical knowledge concerning marijuana's potential benefits and risks has accumulated largely through its widespread use. As mentioned in the previous chapter, a recent poll indicates that approximately one in three Americans over age 12 have tried marijuana or hashish at least once, although only about one in 20 currently use these drugs.

Medical scientists know far more about marijuana's adverse effects than about its ability to relieve specific symptoms, mainly because of the difficulties of conducting clinical research on marijuana. In addition to securing financial support for their research, medical scientists who study marijuana must demonstrate their compliance with a multitude of federal and state regulations before carrying out their investigations (see Chapter 11). Thus, despite recent discoveries highlighted in Chapter 2, substantial clinical studies on the medicinal properties of marijuana remain scarce.

Yet clinical experiments must be undertaken to determine whether marijuana-based medicines live up to their promising performance in numerous basic science studies. Before any medication can be approved for sale by the U.S. Food and Drug Administration, it must pass a series of clinical trials to assure that it is both safe and effective. The trials, which are conducted on healthy volunteers and qualified patients, allow scientists to predict how drugs will perform in the general population.

In a well-designed clinical trial, patients are assigned to treatment groups in such a way that any possible biases in outcome are removed. For example, to compare two medications for nausea, the group of patients being treated with each drug should contain people of equivalent age, gender, and health status. Another approach to providing matched samples is the use of a "crossover" design in which all patients receive both the experimental drug and a placebo in random order.

Clinical trials should also be designed to eliminate the effects of both the patients' and the researchers' expectations concerning the results of the trial. Consider the patient who tries an experimental antinausea drug with the expectation that it will work.

She is far more likely to feel relief after taking the medicine than a patient who does not know if the pill she swallowed contains an active compound, a phenomenon known as the placebo effect. Similarly, knowing whether a patient received the drug or a placebo would likely influence a researcher's evaluation of that patient. For these reasons many clinical studies are designed to be double blind, that is, neither the patient or the researcher knows what treatment the patient has received.

In addition to well-matched treatment groups and double blinding, a good-quality clinical trial also incorporates controls for other factors unrelated to the drug being tested but that nonetheless may influence the treatment outcome. For example, THC reduces anxiety in some people to the extent that they mistakenly believe their symptoms have improved. Although anxiety reduction may be a valuable form of treatment for some patients, it also interferes with attempts to determine whether THC relieves specific symptoms. Successful clinical trials must therefore eliminate this influence—for example, by comparing the effect of THC on a particular symptom with that of a drug known to reduce anxiety but not the specific symptom being studied.

While double-blind, randomized, controlled clinical trials are the best way to evaluate a drug's effectiveness, such trials are not always feasible. For example, children, women of childbearing age, and the elderly are often excluded from experimental drug trials for safety reasons, yet patients in all of these groups take prescription medications. To get around this problem, medical scientists sometimes conduct single-patient trials in which individuals—including patients from vulnerable populations—are treated sequentially with several different medications or are given alternating doses of an experimental drug and a placebo. Although limited in scope, single-patient trials can permit objective comparisons between treatments.

The next six chapters describe scientists' initial attempts to test the safety and effectiveness of marijuana and cannabinoid drugs in the treatment of human patients. The discussion is limited to research on conditions that marijuana has been most often claimed to help, such as pain, AIDS, cancer, and muscular spasticity. Other sources, particularly recent books by Grinspoon and Bakalar and Mathre,[1] discuss indications for marijuana beyond those described here. Most of these less common uses of medical marijuana, such as in patients with Crohn's disease and asthma, are based on a few anecdotal reports. However, since many different disorders share symptoms such as pain, nausea, and muscle spasms, it is possible that a wide variety of patients may be helped by medicines derived from marijuana.

All of the clinical trials we discuss share a common characteristic: they are intended to test whether marijuana or cannabinoids can improve specific symptoms, *not* whether marijuana-based medicines can cure disease. Although marijuana's potential usefulness appears to be limited entirely to relieving discomfort, preliminary evidence indicates that it can provide relief to at least some patients.

Taken as a whole, the results of both basic research and clinical research on marijuana and cannabinoids suggest a variety of potential applications for marijuana-based medicines. Cannabinoids appear to be especially strong candidates for use in pain relievers, antinausea drugs, and appetite stimulants—or perhaps in broad-spectrum medications designed to treat all of these symptoms simultaneously, as they occur in AIDS patients and people undergoing chemotherapy for cancer. Most encouraging marijuana-related clinical studies reflect the therapeutic potential of a single cannabinoid: THC, the primary psychoactive ingredient in marijuana.

Weaker but still favorable scientific evidence supports the use of cannabinoids to treat muscle spasticity in patients with multiple sclerosis or spinal cord injury. The least promising indications discussed here include movement disorders, epilepsy, and glaucoma; nevertheless, animal experiments on movement disorders appear favorable enough to warrant continued exploration in the clinic.

NOTE

1. Grinspoon L, Bakalar JB. 1997. *Marijuana: The Forbidden Medicine.* New Haven, CT: Yale University Press; Mathre ML, ed. 1997. *Cannabis in Medical Practice.* Jefferson, NC: McFarland.

4

MARIJUANA AND PAIN

Pain is the alarm of disease, the symptom that announces that all is not right with our bodies. Whether due to accident or illness, it is the most common reason that people seek medical assistance. But because pain has many causes, some of which are poorly understood, it is often a vexing problem to treat. There are no truly effective medicines for certain types of pain, and sometimes relief comes only at the expense of debilitating side effects. Thus, the search for new and better pain relievers, perhaps the oldest form of medicine, continues unabated.

Early in that pursuit, people discovered the pain-relieving properties of marijuana. It has since been used to treat a wide variety of painful conditions, from headache to the pain of childbirth. Many of the medical marijuana advocates who spoke at the public sessions held by the IOM—among them cancer and AIDS patients, migraine sufferers, and people with spastic and movement disorders—described how marijuana helped relieve their painful symptoms (see Chapter 2). Because marijuana is used to treat pain under such diverse circumstances and because the IOM team determined that marijuana appears to be a promising source of analgesic medications, the next chapter is devoted to discussing the performance of marijuana and cannabinoids in clinical studies of pain relief.

The nerve signals that our brains interpret as pain originate in receptor-bearing cells that become activated by temperature, touch, movement, or chemical changes in their environment. Pain signals travel to the brain by one of three main pathways, described in Box 4.1. Pain may be acute—short lived and intense—or chronic, persisting for days to years. For acute pain, such as the discomfort that follows surgery, doctors typically prescribe opiates: narcotic drugs derived from, or chemically similar to, opium. For chronic pain, however, opiates rarely bring relief. Even when they are effective, opiates often cause nausea and sedation that become a burden to the long-term user. At the very least, people with chronic pain develop tolerance to opiates over months or years and so must continually increase their dosage. Clearly, better pain medications would be welcome. Might marijuana be a source of these sought-after drugs?

Box 4.1
Types of Pain

Pain signals arise and travel to the brain by one of three main pathways, each of which produces different pain sensations:

• *Somatic pain* is the feeling most people imagine when they think about pain: a message sent by receptors located throughout the body whenever injury occurs. Somatic pain signals travel to the brain via peripheral nerves, and are typically experienced as a constant, dull ache in the injured region.

• *Visceral pain* occurs when tissues or organs in the abdominal cavity become stretched or otherwise disturbed due to disease or injury. Pain signals issue from a specific class of receptors present in the gut, producing feelings of pressure deep within the abdomen. Visceral pain often seems to be coming from a different part of the body than its actual source, a phenomenon known as referred pain.

• *Neuropathic pain* occurs when nerves themselves sustain injury. It is often experienced as a burning sensation that can occur in response to even a gentle touch. Neuropathic pain does not usually respond to narcotic painkillers, which relieve many other types of pain. Antidepressant or anticonvulsant drugs, as well as certain surgical procedures, may improve some cases of neuropathy.

Cannabinoids have shown significant promise in basic experiments on pain. Peripheral nerves that detect pain sensations contain abundant receptors for cannabinoids, and cannabinoids appear to block peripheral nerve pain in experimental animals. Even more encouraging, basic studies suggest that opiates and cannabinoids suppress pain through different mechanisms. If that is the case, marijuana-based medicines could perhaps be combined with opiates to boost their pain-relieving power while limiting their side effects.

But because of the ethical and logistical difficulties of conducting pain experiments on human volunteers, marijuana's potential to relieve pain has yet to be conclusively confirmed in the clinic. Only a few such studies have been conducted and only one since 1981. Most tested the ability of cannabinoids to relieve chronic pain in people with cancer or acute pain following surgery or injury. Unfortunately, few of these studies are directly comparable because the methods used to conduct them varied greatly and in some cases appear to have been less than scientifically sound. However, after critically reviewing existing research on THC and pain relief, the IOM team concluded that cannabinoids can provide mild to moderate relief from pain, on a par with codeine. The IOM team also determined that the body's own cannabinoid system likely plays a natural role in pain control.

By contrast, some clinical studies not only have failed to demonstrate that THC relieves pain but have also found that the drug has the opposite effect. In these experiments, volunteers who experienced painful shocks, heat, or pressure from a tourniquet reported that THC actually increased their sensitivity to pain.[1] Another clinical study found that THC merely failed to relieve pain induced by either electrical shock or pressure, but the experiment was flawed in two respects.[2] First, the researchers measured responses to extremes of pain, rather than to more typically painful sensations. Participants were exposed to shocks or pressure over a range of intensities but were only asked to note when they first felt pain and the maximum intensity of pain they could withstand. Since most people take medication for moderate pain, it would have been more useful to evaluate the ability of THC to relieve pain between the extremes that were actually measured (researchers commonly do this by asking participants to use a numerical scale to rate the pain they feel under various conditions). The second problem with this study is that the researchers failed to demonstrate that other painkillers could work under their experimental conditions. Without this standard of comparison, the results on THC have little meaning. They may conflict with those of other studies simply because of the methods the researchers used.

Design flaws also compromise a study that tested smoked marijuana's ability to relieve heat-induced pain in human volunteers. In this experiment, habitual marijuana users were hospitalized and allowed free access to marijuana cigarettes for a period of four weeks. During this time, volunteers consumed an average of four to 17 marijuana cigarettes per day and were tested periodically to gauge their response to painful heat applied to the skin. But since these tests were only performed "approximately every one to two weeks," it is quite likely that the participants had already developed tolerance to the pain-relieving effects of THC by the time the tests were performed. It is therefore not surprising that THC failed to relieve pain under these conditions.

Two studies have examined the effectiveness of THC and levonantradol, a synthetic compound similar to THC, in relieving acute postoperative pain. In the first, volunteers who each had four molars extracted on separate occasions received the local anesthetic lidocaine plus one of the following treatments, given intravenously, with each successive tooth extraction: two different concentrations of THC, the sedative tranquilizer diazepam (Valium), and a placebo. Twenty-four hours after surgery the patients were asked to rate how much pain they felt during the procedure. Based on these ratings the researchers concluded that THC had no effect on surgical pain. There are several reasons to question this conclusion, however. Most importantly, the scientists once again failed to check whether another pain reliever, rather than a sedative, would have fared better than THC in the test. Lidocaine almost certainly diminished the patients' perceptions of pain, which were further compromised because they were not reported until 24 hours after surgery.[3]

The study on levonantradol is less problematic. Researchers gave the drug by intramuscular injection to 56 volunteers 24 to 36 hours after they were treated for injuries or underwent surgery.

To eliminate the possibility that prior drug exposure would influence the patients' experience, the researchers did not test people who had a history of drug abuse or addiction or those who were taking prescription drugs that might interfere with their ability to perceive pain. On average, the researchers reported, patients who received levonantradol after surgery experienced significantly greater pain relief than those who got the placebo. The extent to which patients varied in their response to the drug is not clear, however. The authors do not reveal whether all patients who took the THC analog felt its effects to some extent or whether some people obtained great relief while others found it had little or no effect on their postoperative pain.[4]

The most encouraging—and believable—clinical studies of cannabinoids focus on chronic pain in cancer patients. Cancer causes pain in a variety of ways, including inflammation, nerve injury, and the invasion of bone and other sensitive tissue by growing tumors. Cancer pain tends to be severe, persistent, and resistant to treatment with opiate painkillers. For this reason, researchers hope to discover pain relievers that act on the body in a different way than opiates do.

In one such study, 10 patients with advanced cancer received THC pills in four different doses as well as a placebo. Each patient received the entire range of pills, which were identical in appearance, over successive days. On days when patients received the two highest doses—15 and 20 milligrams of the drug, as compared with 0, 5, or 10 milligrams—they reported significant pain relief. (By comparison, when patients take Marinol for AIDS wasting, an approved indication, they commonly take it in 5-milligram doses, with a maximum dosage of 20 milligrams per day. Marijuana cigarettes contain highly variable amounts of THC, typically between 30 and 150 milligrams, but much of that THC is lost in uninhaled smoke.) The study did not, unfortunately, compare THC with any other painkiller.[5]

Although they reported feeling less pain, patients who received the highest dose of THC in this study were also heavily sedated. They appeared dreamy and immobile; their thoughts were disorganized and they described feelings of unreality. Moreover, during the process of selecting patients to participate in the study, five of 36 volunteers became intensely anxious after receiving 10 to 20 milligrams of THC and as a result were excluded from the experiment. If this experiment is any indication, THC's side effects—though somewhat different—are as problematic as those of opiates.

Interestingly, during this study none of the patients experienced nausea or vomiting and more than half reported that their appetite increased, which suggests that oral THC acted as an antiemetic and an appetite stimulant, as well as a pain reliever. The authors also noted that some patients who appeared calmer after taking THC reported that it had not relieved their pain; other patients said that while their pain remained the same it bothered them less. These impressions resemble several anecdotal reports from marijuana users, who told the IOM team that marijuana did not take away their pain but helped them cope with their discomfort.

In a subsequent study the same researchers compared the effects of a single potent dose of THC with that of a relatively weak narcotic pain reliever, codeine. They found that 10 milligrams of THC gave the same pain relief as a 60-milligram (moderately strong) dose of codeine and that 20 milligrams of THC worked as well as 120 milligrams of codeine. The two drugs produced similar side effects, but THC appeared to be more sedating than codeine. On the other hand, patients tended to have a greater sense of well-being and less anxiety after taking THC than they did under the influence of codeine.[6]

Another group of researchers compared two conventional painkillers, codeine and secobarbital (a short-acting barbiturate), with a synthetic compound similar to THC. This THC analog had previously been shown to block pain in animals, so it was being tested for its ability to relieve moderate to severe pain in cancer patients. Both comparisons were conducted in cancer patients who suffered moderate to severe pain. In one trial 30 such patients were given three different treatments, in random order, on consecutive days: a moderately strong dose of codeine, a standard dose of the experimental cannabinoid, and a placebo. Patients then rated the intensity of their pain on a three-point scale (none, slight, moderate) every hour for six hours. The second trial, which compared the cannabinoid with secobarbital in 15 patients, followed the same procedure. On average, participants found that the THC analog relieved mild, moderate, and severe pain as well as the codeine and better than the secobarbital.[7]

In addition to the clinical trials already discussed, a handful of case studies and surveys have addressed the ability of marijuana or cannabinoids to relieve pain. The case studies are generally unconvincing, but survey responses suggest that marijuana—and by extension cannabinoids—can ease certain chronic pain syndromes. For example, in a recent survey of more than 100 regular marijuana users with multiple sclerosis, nearly every participant reported that marijuana helped relieve spasticity and limb pain (see Chapter 7).[8] Likewise, many paraplegic patients interviewed in an earlier survey stated that smoking marijuana relieved phantom limb pain and headache.[9]

Similar anecdotal evidence has accumulated for the treatment of migraine headaches with marijuana, and marijuana is often mentioned as a "cure" for migraines. Yet the IOM team located only one scientific report on that subject published since 1975. It consists of a description of three cases in which people suffered migraines after quitting their daily marijuana habits.[10] This is hardly convincing evidence that marijuana relieves migraine pain, since it is equally likely that the headaches were caused by withdrawal from the drug. Exploring the possibility of using marijuana-based medicines to relieve migraine pain will require rigorous clinical experiments designed to control for factors that can bias the results.

A possible link between cannabinoids and migraine has been revealed, however, in studies of cannabinoid receptors in the brain. These receptors occur in abundance in the periaqueductal gray (PAG) region, an area where migraines are suspected to arise. But it remains to be determined what effect cannabinoids exert on the PAG and whether they might prevent migraines from occurring. Such research would be worth doing since the best medicine currently available for migraines, sumatriptan (Imitrex), fails to provide complete relief for more than one in four of the patients who use it. An estimated 11 million people in the United States suffer from moderate to severe migraines.

Much of what medical scientists have learned about marijuana's pain-relieving potential warrants further study, according to the IOM team. A logical next step in basic research would be to determine whether existing cannabinoids could be modified to retain their analgesic properties while reducing or removing unwanted side effects such as amnesia and sedation. But some of those side effects may make marijuana an especially useful pain reliever. Cannabinoids appear to reduce nausea, vomiting, and appetite loss as well as pain. And the euphoric lift that attracts recreational users to marijuana could benefit people with anxiety-producing disorders such as AIDS or cancer. In fact, for that reason the IOM team recommended that researchers undertake clinical studies of cannabinoid medications among cancer patients on chemotherapy and AIDS patients suffering from wasting or significant pain. The IOM also recommended that the following groups of patients be included in such studies:

• Surgical patients. In this case, cannabinoids should be administered along with opiates to determine whether cannabinoids reduce the nausea and vomiting associated with opiate painkillers.
• Patients with spinal cord injury or other pain caused by nerve damage.
• Patients with chronic pain who also suffer from insomnia.

All of the above patients are currently treated with opiate drugs, which produce tolerance and dependence as well as undesirable side effects. Could lower doses of opiates give these patients the same degree of relief when supplemented with cannabinoids? The answer lies in carefully conducted clinical experiments. Clinical trials could also determine whether THC is the sole—and, if not, the best—pain-relieving compound in marijuana. If additional cannabinoids relieve pain, researchers must then consider which cannabinoids or combinations thereof work best.

Although there has been very little clinical pain research on marijuana, the findings support positive results from animal and other basic experiments. Further clinical research appears to be well worth pursuing if it leads to a new class of drugs to complement existing painkillers or medications that could simultaneously relieve pain and nausea or appetite loss. The latter would be especially useful to people with AIDS and cancer, as described in the next two chapters.

But these future prospects offer little comfort to people with chronic pain that defies conventional treatments. Accordingly, the IOM researchers recommended the creation of an individual clinical trial program that would allow such patients to smoke marijuana under carefully controlled conditions for a limited period of time. Note that this is *not* the same as reopening the marijuana Compassionate Use Program that was closed in 1991 (see Chapter 11). As described in the IOM report, individual trials would be used to gather information to help develop alternative delivery methods for cannabinoid medications. Participants, who would be fully informed of their status as experimental subjects and the harms inherent in using smoking as a delivery system, would have their condition documented while they continued using marijuana. By analyzing the results of such trials, medical scientists could significantly increase their knowledge of both the positive and the negative effects of medical marijuana use.

NOTES

1. Institute of Medicine. 1999. *Marijuana and Medicine: Assessing the Science Base*. Washington, DC: National Academy Press, p. 141.

2. Raft D, Gregg J, Ghia J, Harris L. 1977. "Effects of intravenous tetrahydrocannabinol on experimental and surgical pain: Psychological correlates of the analgesic response." *Clinical Pharmacology and Therapeutics* 21:26-33.

3. Ibid.

4. Jain AK, Ryan JR, McMahon FG, Smith G. 1981. "Evaluation of intramuscular levonantradol and placebo in acute postoperative pain." *Journal of Clinical Pharmacology* 21:320S-326S.

5. Noyes R Jr, Brunk SF, Baram DA, Canter A. 1975a. "Analgesic effect of delta-9-tetracannabinol." *Journal of Clinical Pharmacology* 15:139-143.

6. Noyes R Jr, Brunk SF, Baram DA, Canter A. 1975b. "Analgesic effect of delta-9-tetracannabinol and codeine." *Clinical Pharmacology and Therapeutics* 18:84-89.

7. Staquet M, Gantt C, Machin D. 1978. "Effect of a nitrogen analog of tetrahydrocannabinol on cancer pain." *Clinical Pharmacology and Therapeutics* 23:397-401.

8. Consroe P, Musty R, Rein J, Tillery W, Pertwee RG. 1997. "The perceived effects of smoked cannabis on patients with multiple sclerosis." *European Neurology* 38:44-48.

9. Dunn M and Davis R. 1974. "The perceived effects of marijuana on spinal cord injured males." *Paraplegia* 12:175.

10. El-Mallakh RS. 1987. "Marijuana and migraine." *Headache* 27:442-443.

5

MARIJUANA AND AIDS

Although no comprehensive surveys have been conducted on medical marijuana users in the United States, small-scale polls indicate that most are seeking relief from symptoms of AIDS. For example, each of the three California cannabis buyers' clubs—organizations that provide marijuana to patients—visited by the IOM team reported that more than 60 percent of their members requested the drug for AIDS treatment.

Age is often cited as the reason why such a large proportion of medical marijuana users in the United States are people with AIDS (this is not the case elsewhere; in Great Britain, for example, multiple sclerosis appears to predominate among medical marijuana users). Because HIV has disproportionately infected members of a generation that grew up experimenting with marijuana, so the theory goes, AIDS patients tend to be comparatively willing to use it as a medicine. By contrast, cancer patients, who are on average older and thus less likely to have tried marijuana, are far less inclined to seek it out. If this reasoning is correct, increasing numbers of cancer patients should turn to medical marijuana as the baby boom generation ages.

Another factor also may contribute to the popularity of medicinal marijuana among people with AIDS: the drug's purported ability to soothe a variety of debilitating symptoms. Many such patients echo the comments of the HIV-positive man cited in

Chapter 2 who claimed that marijuana calmed his stomach after taking medication, stimulated his appetite, eased his pain, and lifted his mood.

Because HIV attacks the immune system, it wreaks havoc throughout the body. Besides providing a foothold for opportunistic infection and cancer, the virus also triggers a potentially lethal wasting syndrome, painful nerve damage, and dementia. Finally, in addition to the physical discomforts inflicted by HIV, many people with AIDS also struggle with depression and anxiety. Marijuana, some patients say, eases all of these problems and more.

Nausea and Vomiting

Even the recent success of combination therapy—which, by keeping HIV in check, has transformed AIDS from a terminal illness to a chronic disorder—has a downside. The very drugs that give people with HIV a future can make their day-to-day life miserable. As this 41-year-old Virginia theater technician told the IOM team:

> Thirteen years ago I found out that I was HIV-positive. Since then I have taken AZT, ddI, d4T, Crixivan, Viracept, Viramune, Bactrim, Megace, and others. All these drugs have two things in common: they gave me hope and they also made me sick. Nausea, diarrhea, fatigue, vomiting, and loss of appetite became a way of life for me.
>
> After three years of these side effects ruling my life, a doctor suggested a simple and effective way to deal with many of them. This remedy kept me from slowly starving to death, as I had seen many of my friends do. It helped me rejoin the human race as a responsible, productive citizen. It also made me a criminal, something I have never been before. This remedy, of course, is medical marijuana.

Like this man, increasing numbers of AIDS patients appear to be using marijuana to counteract the side effects of prescribed medicines as well as to treat disease symptoms. In particular, those who take highly effective antiviral drugs called protease inhibitors often suffer from nausea and vomiting similar to that experienced by cancer patients during chemotherapy.

Just how effectively marijuana and cannabinoids reduce the

nausea and vomiting brought on by AIDS medications remains to be determined in the clinic. Research on marijuana's antinausea properties has focused on chemotherapy-induced emesis (vomiting) in cancer patients and is discussed in depth in the next chapter. Several different types of antiemetic drugs (including substituted benazamides, serotonin receptor antagonists, and corticosteroids) have been used successfully by both AIDS patients and cancer patients, so there is reason to believe that cannabinoids could help both groups. On the other hand, clinical studies indicate that marijuana and THC do not control nausea and vomiting as effectively as do other medications.

Since a wide variety of factors influence emesis and each person responds to them differently, it is possible that certain patients would get better relief from marijuana-based medicines than from conventional treatments. That this is the case remains to be substantiated by controlled studies. In the meantime, some people with AIDS who take THC in the form of dronabinol (Marinol) to combat weight loss may also find that it reduces their feelings of nausea. AIDS patients who took the drug in a four-week clinical study showed a trend toward decreased nausea compared with those who took a placebo, as well as a significant increase in appetite.[1]

AIDS WASTING SYNDROME

While both nausea and appetite loss play a role in wasting, the latter is the primary reason AIDS patients take Marinol. Weight loss is one of two indications for which the U.S. Food and Drug Administration has approved the drug for sale (the other is nausea and vomiting associated with cancer chemotherapy). For people with HIV, loss of as little as 5 percent of their body weight appears to be life threatening. Death from wasting generally occurs when patients drop to more than one-third below their ideal weight.

The Centers for Disease Control and Prevention defines AIDS wasting syndrome as the involuntary loss of more than 10 percent of body weight, accompanied by diarrhea or fever that lasts more than 30 days and is not attributable to another illness. Wasting occurs through a combination of two different physiological processes, cachexia and starvation. Cachexia (pronounced kah-KEK-see-uh) results from tissue injury and causes a disproportionate loss of lean tissue mass, such as muscle or liver; the same process also occurs during the final stages of cancer. Starvation, by contrast, results from food or nutrient deprivation; it causes a loss of body fat before lean tissues become depleted. While starvation can be cured simply by eating, curing cachexia generally requires controlling the disease that triggered it and artificially stimulating the body's metabolism.

Research indicates that people begin losing muscle and other lean tissues even before developing full-blown AIDS, possibly as a result of the body's response to viral infection. Later, opportunistic infections or ulcers of the mouth, throat, or esophagus make eating difficult. Other infectious organisms cause diarrhea, which reduces nutrient absorption, as does the overgrowth of microbes that naturally inhabit the digestive tract. Depression, fatigue, and poverty may further exacerbate malnutrition in AIDS patients.

Standard therapy for AIDS wasting focuses on stimulating the patient's appetite, usually with the drug megestrol acetate (Megace). Although approved for this purpose, Marinol is prescribed far less often. Clinical studies indicate that Megace stimulates weight gain more effectively than Marinol and that patients get no additional benefit by using the drugs in combination.[2] People who take Megace typically increase their food consumption by about 30 percent, but gain mostly fat, rather than lean tissue or muscle mass. Like Megace, Marinol reverses starvation but has no effect on cachexia. Presumably, the same is true of marijuana.

To date, THC is the only cannabinoid that has been evaluated in the clinic for its ability to stimulate appetite and thereby counteract AIDS wasting. In short-term (six weeks) and long-term (one year) studies, patients who received THC in the form of Marinol tended to experience increased appetite while maintaining a stable weight.[3] In addition, five patients in a preliminary study gained an average of 1 percent body fat after taking the drug for five weeks.[4]

Some patients in these and other studies have experienced unpleasant side effects from the drug, ranging from dry mouth to psychological distress. These problems are exacerbated by the difficulty of fine-tuning the dosage of THC in pill form. Moreover, when taken orally, THC tends to be slow to act and to clear from the body.

For these reasons some AIDS patients—and also some cancer patients who have used Marinol to combat wasting and chemotherapy-induced nausea—report that they prefer smoking marijuana to swallowing THC. Smoking, they say, allows them to inhale just enough of the drug to relieve their symptoms. They also cite "the munchies"—well known among marijuana users and documented in laboratory studies of normal, healthy adults who gained both appetite and weight while using marijuana.[5] Unfortunately, there have been no controlled studies to date on the benefits of marijuana smoking on appetite, weight gain, or body composition among people with HIV. In May 2000, Donald Abrams, a medical researcher at the University of California at San Francisco, completed the first controlled study of the short-term safety of smoked marijuana in HIV patients. The results showed that patients who smoked marijuana for 21 days did not show any increase in the HIV virus during the study period.

Clearly, there is a need for medications that can prevent or restore the loss of lean tissues that occurs during AIDS wasting. Preliminary studies of anabolic compounds such as testosterone or growth hormone appear encouraging. Researchers are also investigating whether inhibitors of cytokines—chemical messengers believed to stimulate the inflammatory process that provokes cachexia—could be used to increase lean body mass. While marijuana derivatives do not appear to reverse cachexia, they could potentially form part of a combination treatment for wasting. For example, cannabinoid drugs might be used to boost patients' food consumption while they undergo physical therapy or take medications designed to increase the proportion of lean tissues in their bodies.

PAIN

In addition to appetite stimulation, marijuana-based medicines may prove helpful in treating a variety of painful symptoms associated with AIDS. In particular, many AIDS patients suffer from neuropathic pain, a burning sensation of the skin that occurs spontaneously or is triggered by even the most gentle touch.

While some AIDS patients report that smoking marijuana relieves neuropathic pain, that claim has not been confirmed by a clinical study. As discussed in the previous chapter, researchers have found THC to be moderately effective in treating cancer pain, which includes neuropathy. These results suggest that THC might also provide relief for AIDS-related pain.

EFFECTS ON MOOD

AIDS exacts a toll not only on the body but also on the emotions. Even patients whose disease is effectively controlled must deal with the side effects of medications and cope with having a chronic illness for the rest of their lives. Few escape feeling bereft or anxious from time to time, feelings that often coincide with depression. But some people with AIDS say that, when they use marijuana to relieve their pain or stimulate their appetite, they also improve their mood.

Distinguishing between the medical use of marijuana to treat anxiety or depressed mood and the recreational pursuit of a "high" is not a simple matter, and some would say no such distinction exists. This is an especially thorny issue among AIDS patients, many of whom discover the drug's medical benefits through recreational experience. But there are also patients who, although they began using marijuana to relieve physical symptoms, have come to appreciate the psychological lift it provides.

How often such appreciation of marijuana's psychological effects leads to dependence or abuse remains to be determined. THC, in the form of Marinol, has been found to produce psychological (as well as physiological) dependence in healthy people. But a recent study concluded that for AIDS and cancer patients euphoria was a "desirable side effect" of treatment with Marinol. The study, conducted at San Francisco's Haight Ashbury Clinic, also found that Marinol has a low potential for abuse by patients and that the drug is rarely, if ever, diverted to the black market.[6]

Not everyone, though, reacts positively to marijuana and its active ingredients. Some—typically those who have never used

marijuana before—have reported that smoking marijuana or taking oral THC made them feel so uncomfortable that they never
wanted to use either drug again. Rather than calming them, marijuana or THC seemed to make these people even more anxious;
they also described feeling dizzy, disconnected from reality, even
psychotic. According to medical marijuana advocates, such patients rarely experience adverse psychological reactions if they
are given adequate guidance about what to expect before using
marijuana for the first time. This claim has not been objectively
tested, however.

The fact that the psychoactive effects of marijuana vary
widely from user to user must be anticipated among the potential side effects of any marijuana-based medicine. Unquestion-
ably, marijuana compromises users' cognitive abilities but it
remains to be determined whether long-term marijuana or cannabinoid use actually causes structural damage to the brain (see
Chapter 3).

REDUCING MARIJUANA'S RISKS

While the possibility of cognitive impairment may deter some
people with HIV from using marijuana-based medicines, this haz-
ard pales in comparison to the health risks incurred by smoking
marijuana. As discussed in Chapter 3, harmful smokeborne
chemicals and contaminants in crude marijuana can represent a
serious danger to anyone with a weakened immune system. Research indicates that people with HIV who regularly smoke marijuana suffer higher rates of opportunistic infections and Kaposi's
sarcoma.

Smoking is a very efficient way to get the active chemicals in
marijuana into the bloodstream, but the long-term damage smoking causes makes it a poor drug delivery system, particularly for
patients with chronic illnesses such as HIV. By comparison, oral
cannabinoid preparations, such as Marinol, are slow acting and
difficult to dose properly. A safe and effective alternative to both
routes might be a smokeless inhaler that delivers cannabinoids in
an easily absorbed aerosol spray. Such devices, which are already
used to administer antihistamines and asthma medications, might

allow people with AIDS and other chronic conditions to benefit from marijuana's active ingredients.

Both anecdotal evidence and scientific research suggest that cannabinoids could soothe a variety of symptoms suffered by AIDS patients: nausea, appetite loss, pain, and anxiety. Although more effective medicines than marijuana already exist to treat these conditions, they are not equally effective for all patients, nor do they offer the broad spectrum of relief that might be obtained from cannabinoid drugs. These will only become available, however, if there is sufficient financial incentive for pharmaceutical companies to produce marijuana-based medicines or if public funding supports similar research and development. The perils and possibilities of these alternatives are explored in Chapter 10.

But what about the immediate needs of AIDS patients who have not found relief except by smoking marijuana? The IOM team suggested that people suffering from chronic conditions, including AIDS wasting, could be treated as participants in single-patient clinical trials, carefully monitored and conducted with institutional approval. Once admitted to such trials, patients would be permitted to smoke marijuana under medical supervision but only after being fully informed of their status as experimental subjects and of the harms inherent in using smoking as a delivery system. Each patient's condition would be closely monitored and carefully documented as long as he or she continued to use marijuana. In this way not only would AIDS patients be assured of receiving the best possible treatment, but their experiences would further medical knowledge of marijuana's risks and benefits.

NOTES

1. Beal JE, Olson RLL, Morales JO, Bellman P, Yangco B, Lefkowitz L, Plasse TF, Shepard KV. 1995. "Dronabinol as a treatment for anorexia associated with weight loss in patients with AIDS." *Journal of Pain and Symptom Management* 10:89-97.

2. Timpone JG, Wright DJ, Li N, Egorin MJ, Enama ME, Mayers J, Galetto G. 1997. "The safety and pharmacokinetics of single-agent and combination therapy with megestrol acetate and dronabinol for the treatment of HIV wasting syndrome." The DATRI 004 Study Group. *AIDS Research and Human Retroviruses* 13:305-315.

3. Beal JE, et al. 1995; Beal JE, Olson R, Lefkowitz L, Laubenstein L, Bellman P, Yangco B, Morales JO, Murphy R, Powderly W, Plasse TF, Mosdell KW, Shepard KV. 1997. "Long-term efficiency and safety of dronabinol for acquired immunodeficiency syndrome-associated anorexia." *Journal of Pain Management* 14:7-14.

4. Struwe M, Kaempfer SH, Geiger CJ, Pavia AT, Plasse TF, Shepard KV, Ries K, Evans TG. 1993. "Effect of dronabinol on nutritional status in HIV infection." *Annals of Pharmacotherapy* 27:827-831.

5. Foltin RW, Fischman MW, Byrne MF. 1988. "Effects of smoked marijuana on food intake and body weight of humans living in a residential laboratory." *Appetite* 11:1-14; Mattes RD, Engelman K, Shaw LM, ElSohly MA. 1994. "Cannabinoids and appetite stimulation." *Pharmacology, Biochemistry and Behavior* 49:187-195.

6. Calhoun SR, Galloway GP, Smith DE. 1998. "Abuse potential of dronabinol (Marinol)." *Journal of Psychoactive Drugs* 30:187-196.

6

MARIJUANA AND CANCER

A
pproximately 30 percent of all Americans will develop cancer in their lifetimes. Although two-thirds will eventually die as a result, many will live with cancer for years beforehand. For this reason, researchers not only seek medicines to prevent and cure the disease but also drugs to make life more comfortable for people with cancer.

Is marijuana such a medicine? Several patients and their relatives—many of whom had no prior experience with the drug—have claimed that it is. They include this woman, an author of a 1992 medical marijuana proposal that served as the basis for California's Proposition 215 (see Chapter 11). At the time she was a member of the California Senior Legislature, an elected body that represents the interests of older Californians. Although she herself has never used the drug, she was convinced to take action by her husband's experience, which she described to the IOM team:

> He started chemo. He was ill. He was sicker from the chemo than he was from the cancer, because he wasn't even aware how bad the cancer was. It was not only in the lung; it was in the liver and pancreas. He was given three months.
>
> The oncologist agreed [that] he could use marijuana. I had to do the back alley bit to get some. The first I got wasn't that effective. When I mentioned it to someone, I got a better grade [of mari-

juana]. Two puffs and my husband would go for chemotherapy with a smile and come home happy. He didn't [need to smoke it] again until the next day.

This man died of his cancer but, according to his wife, using marijuana—a drug he would never have tried otherwise—made his last months bearable.

People with cancer who use marijuana say that it benefits them in several ways: by quelling nausea, suppressing vomiting, increasing appetite, relieving pain, and soothing anxiety. Clinical studies indicate that marijuana does none of these things as well as the best medications available, but marijuana has the apparent advantage of treating several symptoms simultaneously. Medicines based on certain chemicals in marijuana could also be used to complement standard medications or to treat patients for whom such therapies have failed.

Considerable clinical evidence indicates that marijuana could yield a variety of useful medicines, especially for nausea, vomiting, and appetite stimulation. THC, in the form of Marinol (dronabinol), has already been used for more than a decade to treat these symptoms in cancer patients and for several years in AIDS patients as well. But other cannabinoids, or combinations of cannabinoids, may prove to be more effective than THC alone. If so, any pharmaceuticals that result from such discoveries could benefit people with AIDS as well as those living with cancer.

CHEMOTHERAPY-INDUCED NAUSEA AND VOMITING

Nausea and vomiting occur when one of several sensory centers, which are located in the brain and the digestive tract, becomes stimulated (see Figure 6.1). It is possible to become nauseous without vomiting or to vomit without feeling nauseous beforehand. Vomiting (also called emesis) involves a complex coordination of the digestive tract, respiratory muscles, and posture. Because all of these actions can be readily measured, scientists have been able to reconstruct the chain of physiological events that lead to vomiting.

Conversely, little is known about the actual mechanisms that trigger nausea, which appears to result from brain activity alone.

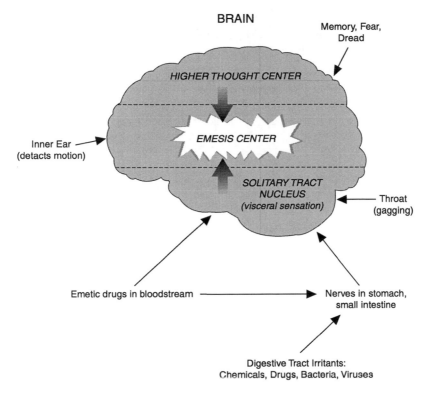

FIGURE 6.1 Emesis pathways. Signals travel to the brain's emesis center, which triggers vomiting, through a variety of routes. Each of these pathways represents a potential site of action for anti-vomiting medications. (Adapted from Bruton LL *The Pharmacological Basis of Therapeutics*, 9th edition. Hardman et al., eds. 1996, p. 929. New York: McGraw-Hill.)

Since nausea lacks any observable action, researchers studying its origins rely on patients' subjective descriptions of their own feelings. As a result of these limitations, most clinical research aimed at relieving the side effects of chemotherapy focuses on the ability of candidate compounds to prevent or curtail vomiting.

Although researchers do not completely understand how chemotherapy agents cause vomiting, they suspect that the drugs or their digestive byproducts stimulate receptors in key sensory cells. Some agents, including cisplatin, cause nearly every patient to vomit repeatedly; others, such as methotrexate, produce this effect in a small minority of chemotherapy patients. Vomiting may begin within a few minutes of treatment, as is the case with the drug mustine, or up to an hour after chemotherapy, as occurs with cisplatin. Most clinical trials of antiemetics—medicines that prevent vomiting—tend to be conducted on patients being treated with cisplatin, because drugs that decrease vomiting following cisplatin treatment are likely to work at least as well as other chemotherapy agents.

Researchers have tested several cannabinoids for their ability to suppress vomiting, including two forms of THC (delta-9 and the less abundant delta-8-THC). Two synthetic cannabinoids (nabilone and levonantradol) that activate the same receptors as THC have also been examined as potential antiemetics. All four compounds have proven mildly effective in preventing vomiting following cancer chemotherapy, as will be described. Two additional clinical studies, also to be discussed, provide evidence that, to a limited extent, smoking marijuana helps suppress chemotherapy-induced emesis.

In clinical comparisons THC tended to reduce chemotherapy-induced vomiting better than a placebo. But few trials have used the same chemotherapy agent among all patients, and some contain substantial flaws. For example, one trial tested THC's effectiveness in patients who received methothrexate—a drug that only occasionally causes vomiting.[1] Some experiments compared the efficacy of THC with prochlorperazine (Compazine), one of the most effective antiemetics available in the 1980s, and found that they were similar. With the advent of more effective medications, such as ondansetron (Zofran) and granisetron (Kytril), both serotonin antagonists, these results carry little weight. Even when administered together, THC and prochlorperazine failed to stop vomiting in two-thirds of patients.[2]

In one particularly well designed study, researchers compared THC with metoclopramide (sold in the United States under various brand names, including Clopra, Maxolon, Octamide PFS, Reclomide, and Reglan), an effective and widely used antiemetic. None of the patients in this study had previously received chemotherapy, so there was no danger that they would vomit simply because they had become conditioned to do so—a reaction that often occurs in people who have undergone several rounds of chemotherapy. Every patient in this study received the same dose of cisplatin; participants were also randomly assigned to receive either THC or metoclopramide. Seventy-three percent of the patients who received THC vomited at least twice following chemotherapy, compared with only 27 percent of the patients who received metoclopramide.[3]

Several additional but less rigorous studies reached similar conclusions: that THC reduces vomiting following chemotherapy, but is not particularly effective in doing so. Nevertheless, the U.S. Food and Drug Administration has approved the drug, in the form of Marinol, for use when chemotherapy-induced nausea and vomiting are not relieved by other antiemetic medications.

Participants in clinical trials of THC have reported several unpleasant side effects, including dry mouth, low blood pressure, sedation, and mood changes. Patients who had no prior experience with marijuana or related drugs were more likely to report psychological discomfort after taking it than those who had tried marijuana previously. On the other hand, advocates of marijuana use for medical purposes maintain that, when such patients receive prior guidance on marijuana's effects, they rarely experience adverse psychological reactions upon using the drug for the first time. Although this claim has not been objectively tested, it may apply equally to the effects of THC, the main psychoactive component in marijuana.

In some clinical trials of THC for antiemesis, patients who underwent the most dramatic mood changes tended to vomit least; other trials found no correlation between THC's psychoactive and antiemetic effects. If they are linked, however, it may be possible to separate the two effects by creating synthetic analogs of the THC molecule. Researchers have found that 11-OH-THC—a breakdown product of THC that forms in the body—is a weaker antiemetic than THC but causes stronger psychological reactions. Perhaps, then, scientists could make additional chemical alterations to the THC molecule to create a chemical analog that controls vomiting better and is less psychoactive than THC.

In fact, such a compound may already exist naturally. Delta-8-THC is a less potent variant of delta-9-THC, the primary psychoactive ingredient in marijuana. In a study of eight children, ages three to 13, delta-8-THC was found to completely block their chemotherapy-induced vomiting. The only side effect reported was irritability in the two youngest children (ages three and one-half and four years).[4]

Of the existing chemical analogs of THC, two have been tested in chemotherapy trials.[5] Nabilone (marketed in the United Kingdom as Cesamet) and levonantradol, neither of which is approved for sale in the United States, fared similarly to THC in these studies. Both were found to be somewhat effective in preventing vomiting following chemotherapy but not as effective as other antiemetics already on the market.

Although many medical marijuana users claim that smoked marijuana controls nausea and vomiting better than oral THC, no rigorous studies that support this contention have yet been published. In a study that directly compared smoked marijuana with THC, researchers found that both prevented vomiting to a similar degree. Only one in four people in this study of 20 patients achieved complete control of chemotherapy-induced vomiting with either drug.[6] Each underwent chemotherapy twice during the trial. During one session, patients smoked a marijuana cigarette and swallowed a placebo pill; at the other session they smoked a placebo cigarette and took a pill containing THC. Patients received the experimental treatments in random order, so approximately half tried marijuana before THC, while the others tried the drugs in the opposite sequence. When asked which form of treatment they preferred, 35 percent of the patients said they favored THC pills, 20 percent chose marijuana, and 45 percent had no preference.

Another preliminary study tested smoked marijuana in cancer patients who were not helped by conventional antiemetic drugs; however, serotonin antagonists—currently considered the most effective antiemetics—were not yet available in 1988 when this study was conducted.[7] Nearly 80 percent of the 56 participants rated marijuana as "moderately effective" or "highly effective," compared with other antiemetics they had previously used. Since this group of patients varied greatly in terms of their chemotheraputic regimen as well as with regard to their prior experience with marijuana, these results must be considered approximate at best.

Nevertheless, it does make sense that inhaling THC in the

form of smoked marijuana would prevent vomiting better than swallowing a pill. If vomiting were severe or began immediately after chemotherapy, oral THC could not stay down long enough to take effect. Smoking also allows patients to take only the drug they want, one puff at a time, thus reducing their risk of unwanted side effects. But the long-term harms of smoking outweigh its benefits for all but the terminally ill, the IOM team concluded. Instead, they recommended the development and testing of a rapid-onset method of delivering THC, such as an inhaler. Similar devices are now used to administer medicine for asthma and other respiratory disorders and are being developed to deliver pain medication.

MALNUTRITION

Wasting and appetite loss affect most cancer patients. At best these conditions diminish quality of life; at worst they hasten death. Depending on the type of cancer, 50 to 80 percent of patients will develop cachexia, a disproportionate loss of lean body tissue. Cachexia occurs most often during the final stages of advanced pancreatic, lung, and prostate cancers. Proteins called cytokines, produced by the immune system in response to the tumor, appear to stimulate this wasting process.

Cachexia also occurs as a result of HIV infection (see Chapter 5), and both cancer and AIDS patients currently receive similar treatments for the condition. Standard therapies for cachexia include intravenous or tube feeding as well as treatment with megestrol acetate (Megace), an appetite stimulant. If the latter causes patients to gain weight, however, it is mostly in the form of fat—not the lean tissue they would have lost through cachexia.

Marijuana is renowned for its ability to stimulate the appetite, otherwise known as "having the munchies." This effect is due in large part to the action of THC, which has been confirmed in several studies.[8] For example, cancer patients who took THC in the form of dronabinol tended to experience a slowing of weight loss and an increase in appetite.[9] A study of AIDS patients, however, indicated that megestrol acetate stimulated weight gain more effectively than THC; when used in combination, the two drugs failed to augment each other's effects.[10]

Both megestrol acetate and dronabinol produce troublesome side effects in some patients. The former can cause hyperglycemia and hypertension; the latter can cause dizziness and lethargy. Because of these drawbacks, medical researchers are pursuing better treatments for cachexia. One promising class of compounds includes agents that can block the actions of the cytokines that promote wasting. Some patients might benefit from a combination therapy consisting of a cytokine blocker along with THC, to stimulate appetite and also, perhaps, to reduce nausea, pain (see Chapter 4), and anxiety.

HARDLY A MAGIC BULLET

Taken as a whole, clinical studies on cannabinoids and cancer pain have reached conclusions similar to those of comparable studies on nausea and malnutrition: marijuana-based treatments, while somewhat effective, underperform conventional medications and cause numerous side effects. The main advantage of cannabinoids lies in their potential to relieve several symptoms at once, but this versatility may come at the price of diminished potency.

For example, powerful opiate medications appear to relieve debilitating pain more effectively than cannabinoids. However, since they appear to reinforce the effects of opiates, cannabinoids may be useful as an adjunct to the stronger drugs. Patients who achieve the same relief with lower doses of opiates should also experience fewer narcotic side effects, such as constipation, drowsiness, and slowed breathing. Moreover, cannabinoids may counteract another common side effect of narcotics—nausea.

Nevertheless, most chemotherapy patients probably would not choose marijuana or THC as an antiemetic. Compared with the highly effective agents currently available, marijuana-based versions appear to offer most people only modest relief. In addition, many patients in clinical studies—in contrast to accounts of several patients who spoke at the IOM's public sessions—have found the side effects of marijuana to be intolerable. In particular, patients who have never smoked marijuana tend to react adversely to the drug's mood-altering properties.

But for the small proportion of patients who respond poorly

to conventional antiemetics, cannabinoids may be a useful alternative. And since they appear to suppress nausea and vomiting through different mechanisms than do other antiemetic compounds, cannabinoids may be able to boost the efficacy of superior medications. For these reasons the IOM study team recommended that researchers test the combined effects of cannabinoids and other antiemetics in suppressing nausea and vomiting in patients who respond poorly to standard treatments.

As described earlier, the IOM team also recommended the development of a rapid-onset drug delivery system that could provide the benefits of inhaling cannabinoids without the harmful effects of smoking. In the meantime for the small minority of cancer patients who have found that only smoking marijuana relieves their chemotherapy-induced vomiting, the IOM team concluded that the harmful effects of doing so for a limited time (i.e., during the course of chemotherapy treatment) might be outweighed by the antiemetic benefits. Such patients, the team suggested, should be evaluated on a case-by-case basis. Those who meet the following conditions could then be provided with marijuana for use under close medical supervision:

• Documented evidence confirms that all approved medications have failed to provide relief.
• There is reasonable expectation that the patient's symptoms could be relieved by inhaling cannabinoids.
• Patients are treated under medical supervision and their treatment is assessed for effectiveness.
• All such treatments are overseen by an institutional review board, such as is required for all federally funded research involving human subjects. (Institutional review boards consist of scientists with expertise in the areas being researched but who are not involved in the specific study being evaluated. The review board approves studies only after determining that the research will not violate the rights and welfare of human participants.)

For the terminally ill, the dangers of smoking are irrelevant. From a strictly medical standpoint—social consequences notwithstanding—there is no reason to deny marijuana to a dying person. But this step should be seen for what it is—a last resort. Clinical evidence shows that existing treatments for pain, nausea, and malnutrition outperform marijuana in the vast majority of patients. To substitute marijuana for a more effective drug is to practice bad medicine.

NOTES

1. Chang AE, Shiling DJ, Stillman RC, et al. 1979. "Delta-9-tetrahydrocannabinol as an antiemetic in patients receiving high-dose methotrexate: A prospective, randomized evaluation." *Annals of Internal Medicine* 91:819-824.

2. Frytak S, Moertel CF, O'Fallon J, et al. 1979. "Delta-9-tetrahydrocannabinol as an antiemetic in patients treated with cancer chemotherapy: A double comparison with prochlorperazine and a placebo." *Annals of Internal Medicine* 91:825-830.

3. Gralla RJ, Tyson LB, Borden LB, et al. 1984. "Antiemetic therapy: A review of recent studies and a report of a random assignment trial comparing metoclopramide with delta-9-tetrahydrocannabinol." *Cancer Treatment Reports* 68:163-172.

4. Abrahamov A, Abrahamov A, Mechoulam R. 1995. "An efficient new cannabinoid antiemetic in pediatric oncology." *Life Sciences* 56:2097-2102.

5. Steele N, Gralla RJ, Braun DW Jr. 1980. "Double-blind comparison of the antiemetic effects of nabilone and prochlorperazine on chemotherapy-induced emesis." *Cancer Treatment Report* 64:219-224; Tyson LB, Gralla RJ, Clark RA, et al. 1985. "Phase I trial of levonantradol in chemotherapy-induced emesis." *American Journal of Clinical Oncology* 8:528-532.

6. Levitt M, Faiman C, Hawks R, et al. 1984. "Randomized double-blind comparison of delta-9-THC and marijuana as chemotherapy antiemetics." *Proceedings of the American Society for Clinical Oncology* 3:91.

7. Vinciguerra V, Moore T, Brennan E. 1988. "Inhalation of marijuana as an antiemetic for cancer chemotherapy." *New York State Journal of Medicine* 88:525-527.

8. Gorter R. 1991. "Management of anorexia-cachexia associated with cancer and HIV infection." *Oncology* (Suppl.) 5:13-17; Beal JE, Olson RLL, Morales JO, Bellman P, Yangco B, Lefkowitz L, Plasse TF, Shepard KV. 1995. "Dronabinol as a treatment for anorexia associated with weight loss in patients with AIDS." *Journal of Pain and Symptom Management* 10:89-97; Beal JE, Olson R, Lefkowitz L, Laubenstein L, Bellman P, Yangco B, Morales JO, Murphy R, Powderly W, Plasse TF, Mosdell KW, Shepard KV. 1997. "Long-term efficiency and safety of dronabinol for acquired immunodeficiency syndrome-associated anorexia." *Journal of Pain Management* 14:7-14.

9. Plasse TF, Gorter RW, Krasnow SH, Maontague L, Shepard KV, Wadleigh RG. 1991. "Recent clinical experience with dronabinol." *Pharmacology, Biochemistry, and Behavior* 40:665-670.

10. Timpone JG, Wright DJ, Li N, Egorin MJ, Enama ME, Mayers J, Galetto G. 1997. "The safety and pharmacokinetics of single-agent and combination therapy with megestrol acetate and dronabinol for the treatment of HIV wasting syndrome." The DATRI 004 Study Group. *AIDS Research and Human Retroviruses* 13:305-315.

7

MARIJUANA AND
MUSCLE SPASTICITY

C oping with stiff, aching, cramping muscles is a way of life for most of the 2.5 million people in the world who have multiple sclerosis. Many of the 15 million people with spinal cord injuries also suffer from the same symptoms, which cause pain, limit movement, and rob people of needed sleep. Although several conventional medications can reduce these patients' discomfort, taking them rarely provides complete relief. Often the drugs cause weakness, drowsiness, and other side effects that some patients find intolerable.

Given this outlook, it is not hard to understand why some people with multiple sclerosis and spinal cord injuries have sought relief through marijuana. Several such patients told the IOM team that their muscle spasms decreased after smoking marijuana (see Chapter 2). Some also said they valued the drug because it relieved nausea or helped them sleep. Likewise, in a 1982 survey of people with spinal cord injuries, 21 of 43 respondents reported that marijuana reduced muscle spasticity[1] (a condition in which muscles tense reflexively and resist stretching), while nearly every participant in a 1997 survey of 112 regular marijuana users with multiple sclerosis replied that the drug lessened both pain and spasticity.[2] This is not to say that most people with multiple sclerosis find relief with marijuana but only that the marijuana users among them do.

Animal research, too, suggests that marijuana calms muscle spasticity. Spasms are thought to originate in areas of the brain that control movement, including several sites with abundant cannabinoid receptors. In one experiment, researchers found that rodents became more animated under the influence of small amounts of cannabinoids but less active when they received larger doses. Many marijuana users also note that the drug affects movement, making their bodies sway and their hands unsteady. The exact mechanism(s) by which cannabinoids exert these effects remains unknown.

Despite these suggestive findings and the depth of anecdotal evidence, marijuana's antispasmodic properties remain largely untested in the clinic. The few existing reports are extremely limited in scope; for example, none of the studies discussed in this chapter included more than 13 patients, and some were conducted on a single patient. Also, in several cases the patients' subjective evaluations of improvement contrasted with objective measures of their physical performance. Still, the lack of good universally effective medicine for muscle spasticity is a compelling reason to continue exploring cannabinoid drugs in the clinic.

MULTIPLE SCLEROSIS

Multiple sclerosis (or MS) is a progressive disease of the nervous system with no known cure. It appears to result from a malfunction of the immune system, which inflames nerves in the brain, brain stem, and spinal cord. Specifically, the disease destroys the protective coating called myelin that sheaths the neural fibers like insulation on electrical wire. Without an intact myelin layer, nerve cells lose some or all of their ability to transmit impulses. This situation produces an array of symptoms, including fatigue, depression, vertigo, blindness, incontinence, and loss of voluntary muscle control, as well as muscle spasticity. MS is characterized by scarring—"sclerosis"—that occurs in the white matter of the central nervous system after nerves and myelin are lost.

Approximately 90 percent of MS patients develop spasticity. Some people experience this condition merely as muscle stiffness; others endure constant ache, cramps, or involuntary muscle contractions (spasms) that are both painful and debilitating. These spasms often affect the legs and can disrupt sleep. Most people with MS experience intermittent "attacks" of spasticity that become increasingly disabling the longer they have the disease. In the worst cases, patients become partially or even completely paralyzed.

The drugs most commonly prescribed to treat the symptoms of MS include baclofen (Lioresal) and tizanidine (Zanaflex) which relieve both spasticity and muscle spasms but often only partially and sometimes not at all. Both are sedatives, so they cause drowsiness; additional side effects include dry mouth and muscle weakness. The latter is especially problematic for people with MS, whose muscles get weaker as the disease progresses.

Both marijuana and THC have been tested for their ability to relieve spasticity in small but rigorous clinical studies. One double-blind experiment (see Introduction to Part II for an explanation of double-blind methods) included both MS patients and unaffected individuals.[3] Before and after smoking a single marijuana cigarette that contained approximately 15 milligrams of THC—enough to make most people feel "high" and to impair their motor control—patients were videotaped as they stood on a platform that slid back and forth at unpredictable times. The researchers then measured participants' shoulder movements as an index for how well they kept their balance.

Participants with MS often thought that their symptoms had improved after smoking marijuana. But while their spasticity may indeed have decreased (it was not measured), their posture and balance were actually impaired; this was also the case with the 10 participants who did not have MS. The MS patients had greater difficulty maintaining their balance before smoking and were more negatively affected by marijuana than the healthy participants.

While the fact that every MS patient in the previous study experienced relief is intriguing, it does not constitute strong evidence that marijuana relieves spasticity because marijuana-induced euphoria or pain relief might decrease patients' perceptions of muscle stiffness or spasticity. The same is true of respondents to the surveys described earlier. Moreover, surveys cannot measure the degree to which respondents feel better simply because they expect to do so. Such placebo effects are significant; for example, in controlled trials of pain medications, as many as 30 percent of the participants who received a placebo reported feeling relief. This does not mean that placebo effects are not "real." It is possible that the psychological effects of taking a placebo drug cause physiological changes in the brain. But it does mean that the effects are not directly due to the medication being tested.

THC's effects on spasticity were tested in three separate clinical studies, which together enrolled a total of 30 MS patients.[4] All three were open trials in which participants knew they would be receiving THC. Perhaps not surprisingly, most of the patients—or in one case the investigators who examined them—reported that treatment with THC improved their symptoms (see Figure 7.1). The drug was not effective for all patients, however, and frequently caused unpleasant side effects.

Objective measurements of patients' symptoms in these studies were often at odds with their subjective reports. In one study researchers measured muscle tremor with a mechanical device, which showed detectable change in only two of eight patients, seven of whom had reported improved symptoms. [5] In another study standardized physician's measures showed that treatment with THC had not produced any changes in spasticity despite reports of reduced spasticity by 11 of 13 patients.[6] It may be that the measuring techniques used in both studies were not sensitive enough to detect subtle improvements. It is also possible that patients' reports of symptom improvement were influenced by placebo effects or by effects of THC, such as anxiety reduction, that are only indirectly related to spasticity. Neither possibility can be ruled out due to the small size of these studies.

In addition to these experiments on THC, a single patient who tested the THC analog nabilone—a synthetic compound that activates the same cellular receptors as THC—also reported an improvement in spasticity as well as in other MS symptoms (see Figure 7.2).[7]

These clinical results are considerably less dramatic than survey and anecdotal reports of marijuana's effectiveness in relieving muscle spasms. It is possible, however, that a series of larger, better-designed clinical trials would produce stronger evidence in favor of marijuana-based medicines for MS. At this writing

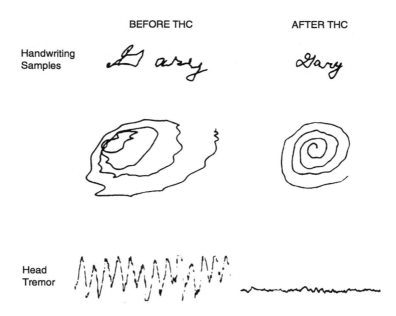

FIGURE 7.1 Effect of THC on tremor caused by multiple sclerosis. In this experiment, a 30-year-old man with multiple sclerosis who suffered from a disabling tremor was treated with 5 milligrams of THC. Researchers compared the man's handwriting and head movement before, and 90 minutes after, receiving the drug. (Reprinted by permission of D.B. Clifford and the *Annals of Neurology*. Tetrahydrocannabinol for tremor in multiple sclerosis. 1983. *Annals of Neurology* 13(6):669-671.)

such studies are in the planning stages in Britain, where a large proportion of medical marijuana users are people with MS. For example, researchers have proposed a clinical trial to compare the effectiveness of three types of treatment for MS: marijuana extract, delivered by inhaler; dronabinol (Marinol); and placebo.

Clinical trials usually require preliminary experiments on animal models of a disease, which enable researchers to predict its effects on humans. With that knowledge scientists can then design trials that accurately measure the ability of the drug to relieve patients' symptoms. Existing animal models mimic some MS symptoms, but so far none have succeeded in duplicating spasticity. But researchers can use the best-available indicator of

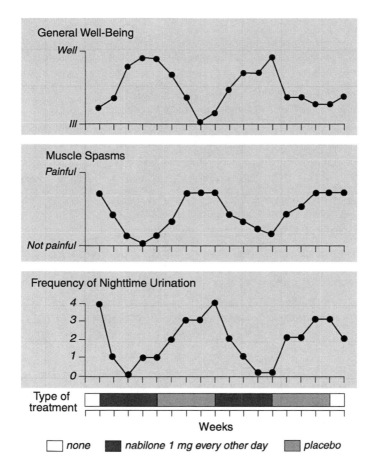

FIGURE 7.2 Effect of nabilone on multiple sclerosis symptoms. This chart shows the results of a trial in which a 45-year-old man with MS received treatments with the THC analog nabilone, alternating with a placebo. While the results suggest that THC might relieve spasticity, the study has several flaws. First, nabilone sedated the patient, which may have caused him to feel some relief; the placebo did not. Second, instead of measuring spasticity, the researchers measured the patient's perception of pain, which may have been relieved without any improvement in spasticity.

Because nighttime urination is not governed by conscious control, improvement in this symptom appears to provide stronger evidence that THC reduced spasticity. On the other hand, it may merely indicate that THC helped the patient sleep better. While intriguing, this single-patient trial does not prove that THC can reliably relieve spasticity.

(Figure used by permission of C.N. Martyn and *The Lancet*. Nabilone in the treatment of multiple sclerosis. *The Lancet* 345(March 4, 1995):579.)

the condition, known as the pendulum test, to study the effectiveness of antispasticity drugs in human subjects.

Participants in this test lie on an examining table with their legs extending over the edge. They let their legs fall, and a video camera records the resulting motion, which is affected by muscle resistance. Computer analysis of the recording enables researchers to determine the degree to which spasticity impeded each patient's movement. Since THC is mildly sedating it is important to distinguish this effect from any actual decrease in spasticity produced by the drug. Researchers could make such a distinction by using the pendulum test to compare THC's effects with those of other mild sedatives, such as benzodiazepines.

If an antispasmodic drug is developed from THC, its sedative effect could prove beneficial to MS patients whose muscle spasms interrupt their sleep. Drowsiness at bedtime might be welcome, and any mood-altering side effects might be less of a problem than when the patient was awake. It is also possible, however, that THC might disrupt normal sleep patterns in some people.

TOWARD BETTER TREATMENTS

While the same physiological process causes spasticity in both MS and spinal cord injury, it produces quite different symptoms in the two diseases. People with MS tend to experience occasional "attacks" of intense pain, stiffness, or muscle spasms at unpredictable intervals, while people with spinal cord injuries experience only minor fluctuations and persistent discomfort. Nevertheless, it is very likely that the same drugs could be adapted to treat the two groups of patients. People with MS and those with spinal cord injury alike would benefit from medications that relieve pain, stiffness, and spasms without muscle weakening, which occurs with the best currently available treatments. Because of the harms associated with long-term marijuana smoking, it should be discouraged as a means of treating chronic conditions such as spinal cord injury or MS.

Whether marijuana could yield useful medicines for spasticity remains to be determined, for the clinical evidence to date is too sparse to accept. But the few positive reports of the ability of THC and nabilone to reduce spasticity, together with numerous anecdotal accounts from marijuana users with MS and spinal cord injuries, suggest that carefully designed clinical trials testing the effects of cannabinoids on muscle spasticity would be worthwhile.

Two factors complicate the design of such trials. First, while MS patients report that marijuana relieves spasticity, it negatively affects their ability to balance, exacerbating another symptom of the disorder. It may be that patients would become tolerant to the balance-impairing effects of cannabinoids relatively quickly yet continue to get relief from spasticity. It might also be possible to separate these effects by creating chemical variants of natural cannabinoids. Second, human trials should rule out any masking or enhancing effect of anxiety reduction due to THC, since anxiety worsens spasticity in many patients.

If THC or a related compound does prove to relieve spasticity, it would make sense for some patients to take the drug orally. In this way patients could take advantage of THC's ability to remain active in the body for several hours. People with spinal cord injury, whose symptoms vary little throughout the day, could get extended relief from a pill taken at bedtime or in the morning. On the other hand, MS patients might find more use for an inhaled form of THC to relieve their more intermittent symptoms. Unlike pills, this delivery method would allow patients to feel the drug's effects quickly and with a minimum of sedation. At nighttime MS patients might actually prefer pills that cause drowsiness as well as relieve spasticity.

People with MS may soon be able to test a cannabinoid inhaler if the previously described British clinical trials receive funding. Additional trials may take place in Canada, where in July 1999 the government issued a request for research proposals to study medical uses of marijuana. While the official announcement did not prescribe specific research topics, it mentioned multiple sclerosis as a possible subject for a clinical trial.

NOTES

1. Malec J, Harvey RF, Cayner JJ. 1982. "Cannabis effect on spasticity in spinal cord injury." *Archives of Physical Medicine and Rehabilitation* 63:116-118.
2. Consroe P, Musty R, Rein J, Tillery W, Pertwee RG. 1997. "The per-

ceived effects of smoked cannabis on patients with multiple sclerosis." *European Neurology* 38:44-48.

3. Greenberg HS, Werness SA, Pugh JE, Andrus RO, Anderson DJ, Domino EF. 1994. "Short-term effects of smoking marijuana on balance in patients with multiple sclerosis and normal volunteers." *Clinical Pharmacology and Therapeutics* 55:324-328.

4. Clifford DB. 1983. "Tetrahydrocannabinol for tremor in multiple sclerosis." *Annals of Neurology* 13:669-671; Petro D and Ellenberger Jr C. 1981. "Treatment of human spasticity with delta-9-tetrahydrocannabinol." *Journal of Clinical Pharmacology* 21:413S-416S; Ungerleider JT, Andrysiak TA, Fairbanks L, Ellison GW, Myers LW. 1987. "Delta-9-THC in the treatment of spasticity associated with multiple sclerosis." *Advances in Alcohol and Substance Abuse* 7:39-50.

5. Clifford DB. 1983.

6. Ungerleider JT, et al. 1987.

7. Martyn CN, Illis LS, Thom J. 1995. "Nabilone treatment of multiple sclerosis." *Lancet* 345:579.

8

MARIJUANA AND
NEUROLOGICAL DISORDERS

W hile frequently touted as a folk remedy for spastic- ity, marijuana is only occasionally mentioned with regard to other neurological disorders. Perhaps people with movement disorders, epilepsy, or Alzheimer's dis- ease derive little benefit from marijuana, but it may also be the case that relatively few patients with these conditions have tried it.

Only a handful of clinical trials have explored the effects of marijuana or cannabinoids on the symptoms of neurological dis- orders other than multiple sclerosis. For the most part these stud- ies are too small to be considered conclusive, and their results are far from promising. Nevertheless, they are worth considering in light of the abundance of cannabinoid receptors in the brain, es- pecially in areas associated with Parkinson's and Huntington's diseases. And since conventional treatments for movement disor- ders, epilepsy, and Alzheimer's disease leave much to be desired, no source of potential remedies should be overlooked.

MOVEMENT DISORDERS

This group of neurological diseases is caused by defects in the basal ganglia, clusters of nerve cells in the brain that control muscular activity. Injury to these regions ultimately affects the motion of muscles in the face, limbs, and trunk. The movement disorders most often discussed as candidates for marijuana-based therapies are dystonias, Huntington's disease, Parkinson's disease and Tourette's syndrome. As a general consideration, it is important to note that stress and anxiety tend to worsen the symptoms of movement disorders. Thus, marijuana's calming effect could be a primary reason why some patients claim that it brings them relief.

Dystonias are a subgroup of movement disorders that share similar symptoms: slow, sustained, involuntary muscle contractions that often cause sufferers to hold their limbs, trunks, or necks in odd positions. They may be confined to one part of the body; for example, spasmodic torticollis affects only the neck, while Meige's syndrome distorts the face. These chronic, slowly progressive disorders are often painful and can cause mild to severe disability. Some dystonias are inherited, while others occur as side effects of certain drugs. Scientists have yet to discover the specific neurological malfunctions that cause dystonias.

Several different drugs are used to treat various forms of dystonia. The most commonly prescribed drugs—benzodiazepines, baclofen, Botulinum toxin, anticholinergic agents, and tetrabenazine—merely relieve the symptoms of dystonia rather than resolving the condition itself. In many cases the relief they provide is incomplete. Baclofen (Lioresal) and benzodiazepines, including diazepam (Valium) and clonazepam (Klonopin, Rivotril), act by reducing the nervous system's ability to stimulate muscle contractions. Both drugs usually make patients drowsy and may also cause a range of additional side effects, including muscle weakness and behavioral problems. Botulinum toxin—a bacterial compound that also causes food poisoning—also blocks muscle stimulation; it produces few side effects but must be injected directly into the affected muscles. Anticholinergic drugs such as trihexyphenidyl (Artane) and diphenhydramine (Benadryl) deactivate muscle contractions; they, too, cause drowsiness and other side effects that can become severe at high doses. Tetrabenazine, although not available in the United States, is a dopamine-depleting compound available in Canada and Europe that is often prescribed for the relief certain types of dystonia.

No controlled study of marijuana in patients with dystonia

has yet been published. Cannabidiol, a chemical component of marijuana (see Chapter 2), was tested in a preliminary open trial in which patients knew they were receiving the experimental drug. The five participants showed only modest improvements, which increased with the amount of drug they received.[1] Better results occurred in a study of an animal model for dystonia—a mutant strain of hamsters—in which researchers tested a synthetic cannabinoid that activates the same cellular receptors as THC. The hamsters exhibited a type of dystonia that produces either sudden spasms of rapid, jerky motions or slow, repetitive writhing movements, both of which decreased under the influence of the cannabinoid.[2]

Besides being a diagnosis in its own right, dystonia is also a symptom of other major movement disorders, including *Huntington's disease*. This inherited disorder usually manifests itself in middle age, continues to worsen, and ultimately leads to death within 15 years of its appearance. Symptoms include rapid, uncontrolled muscle movements (called "chorea," from the Greek word for dance), emotional disturbance and eventually dementia. Patients may take drugs, including reserpine or haloperidol, mainly to control their psychological symptoms. All of these medicines produce adverse side effects, so physicians often wait to prescribe them until a patient's symptoms become severe.

Since anxiety and stress appear to worsen involuntary movements in many patients with Huntington's disease and since marijuana reduces those feelings in most users, some have proposed it as an alternative to existing medications. Animal studies suggest that cannabinoids might suppress choreic movements, presumably by stimulating receptors in the basal ganglia (see Chapter 2). In a preliminary study of four people with Huntington's disease, one patient showed improvement under the influence of cannabidiol.[3] Based on this limited success, researchers attempted a double-blind crossover study (see Introduction to Part II for a discussion of clinical study design) on 15 patients who were not taking medications to inhibit chorea but found that participants' symptoms neither improved nor worsened after treatment with cannabidiol.[4] These results are perhaps to be expected, though, since cannabidiol does *not* bind to the predominant type of cannabinoid receptor (CB_1) on neurons affected by Huntington's disease. THC or other cannabinoids that readily bind CB_1 receptors seem likelier candidates as medications for Huntington's disease, but their effects on patients with the disorder remain unknown.

One of the most devastating movement disorders, *Parkinson's disease*, affects approximately 1 million Americans age 50 and older. Symptoms include tremor, muscular rigidity, instability, and impeded motion (both slowed movement and abrupt stopping in midmovement). The single most effective drug to treat Parkinson's disease, levodopa (L-Dopa, Larodopa, Dopar), has many drawbacks, so physicians tend to reserve it for functionally impaired patients. After several years of use, levodopa tends to wear off quickly after each dose, so patients constantly cycle through phases of mobility and disability. Additional side effects include nausea, hallucination, and confusion. Researchers also suspect that, while levodopa dramatically improves all of the signs and symptoms of Parkinson's disease, its use may accelerate the disease's progress; no clinical evidence confirms this concern.

Because they act on the same neurological pathways that Parkinson's disease disrupts, cannabinoids could in theory be useful in treating the disorder (see Chapter 2). The IOM team found only one published account of a clinical trial of marijuana for Parkinson's disease. The study was prompted by a patient's report that smoking marijuana reduced tremor, but when researchers tested the drug on five additional patients with tremor, they found no evidence of improvement. On the other hand, conventional medications, including levodopa, successfully reduced tremor in all five patients.[5]

Unlike Huntington's and Parkinson's diseases, *Tourette's syndrome* typically appears during childhood. Patients exhibit a variety of rapid, involuntary, repetitive movements and vocalizations, collectively called tics. The causes of Tourette's syndrome are largely unknown but are thought to impair brain areas that convert a person's intent to move into actual movements. Damage to these same areas produces involuntary movement in Huntington's disease and restricts voluntary movement in Parkinson's disease.

Two widely used medications for Tourette's syndrome, pimozide (Orap) and haloperidol (Haldol) inhibit the effects of the neurotransmitter dopamine. Cannabinoids, by contrast, increase dopamine release, so one might predict that cannabinoids would actually exacerbate the symptoms of Tourette's syndrome. Yet four clinical case histories indicate that marijuana use can reduce tics in Tourette's patients. In three of the four cases, however, the investigators suggest that marijuana's anxiety-reducing properties—rather than any specific effect on the neural pathway that produces tics—caused the patients' symptoms to improve.[6]

In summary, while persuasive basic evidence exists for the role of cannabinoids in movement, clinical evidence for their usefulness in relieving the symptoms of movement disorders is lacking. The few existing studies were performed on small numbers of patients and without consideration that marijuana's antianxiety effects might reduce the symptoms in question. Moreover, while there are a few isolated anecdotal reports that marijuana helps patients with these disorders, there are no surveys to suggest that these patients' experiences are at all representative.

Thus, with the possible exception of spasticity in multiple sclerosis, there is little reason to recommend additional clinical trials of marijuana or cannabinoids for movement disorders, the IOM study team concluded. That is not to say that more extensive animal studies will never provide stronger evidence in favor of human trials. But until reliable animal models exist for most movement disorders, such evidence is unlikely to be forthcoming. In the meantime the IOM team recommends conducting double-blind, placebo-controlled clinical trials of individual cannabinoids such as THC—but not smoked marijuana—for the treatment of movement disorders.

The IOM team further specified that these trials should test the effects of cannabinoids on movement alone—that is, the experiments should distinguish cannabinoids' effects on movement from their effects on anxiety or mood. For if cannabinoids merely provide a psychological boost to people with multiple sclerosis, their use would probably not warrant the risk of short-term memory loss, cognitive impairment, and other known side effects. But if cannabinoids directly improve spasticity and other movement-related symptoms, as well as mood, they would offer a uniquely useful treatment. Cannabinoids therefore represent an interesting possibility for treating movement disorders but one that has yet to be proven.

A chronic seizure disorder, epilepsy affects about 2 million Americans and an estimated 30 million people worldwide. Symptoms include recurrent sudden attacks of altered consciousness, convulsions, and other uncontrolled movement, apparently brought on by the simultaneous stimulation of numerous nerve cells. People may become vulnerable to epileptic seizures through a wide variety of possible causes, including physical injury and exposure to chemical toxins.

Some people with epilepsy have partial seizures, which are also known as focal seizures. These disturbances arise in the cerebral cortex, a part of the brain that governs consciousness, movement, and sensation—functions that become temporarily disordered when partial seizures occur. Other people with epilepsy, who develop the condition after sustaining damage to centrally important regions in the brain, experience seizures that affect many aspects of behavior. These generalized seizures may occur as either relatively mild petit mal or violent grand mal events.

A variety of conventional anticonvulsant medications may be used in attempts to control epileptic seizures. Because different drugs work better for different types of seizures, patients must often try several medications before finding the most effective treatment. In general, antiepilepsy drugs suppress seizures completely in about 60 percent of patients and reduce their severity in another 15 percent or so. Many of the remaining 25 percent suffer from a serious underlying brain disease that cannot be relieved through anticonvulsant therapy; others continue to have seizures because they refuse prescribed medication, they use it incorrectly, or their bodies do not reliably absorb the drugs.

Anticonvulsants commonly make people feel drowsy and mentally slow; the drugs may also cause tremor, hair loss, headache, dermatitis, and several other side effects. Nevertheless, most people with epilepsy endure these drawbacks in order to prevent seizures, which can be both physically dangerous and emotionally devastating.

Although some anecdotal accounts—as well as a few reports from small clinical and individual case studies—suggest that marijuana helps control epileptic seizures, no solid evidence supports this assertion.[7] The only relevant controlled study that has been published to date was designed to evaluate whether illicit drug use affected the age at which people with epilepsy had their first seizures. In this study of 600 patients, researchers found that men, but not women, who used marijuana were less prone to develop seizures than men who did not use the drug, suggesting that marijuana provided some sort of protection for men.[8] However, it is also possible that the marijuana-using men in this study tended to be healthier than those who had not used the drug; in other words, their health status influenced their drug use rather than the other way around.

Researchers have also investigated the antiepileptic properties of cannabidiol, which shows little promise. In three controlled trials conducted with patients with both focal and generalized epilepsy, oral doses of cannabidiol failed to lessen the frequency of either type of seizure.[9] Even if cannabidiol had appeared to suppress seizures, however, these trials would have been far too small to prove its effectiveness. Studies of drugs for epilepsy generally require large numbers of patients who must be followed for months, since symptoms are highly variable and tend to occur unpredictably.

Currently, the only biological reason to believe that cannabinoids could suppress epileptic seizures is the abundance of CB_1 receptors in some of the regions of the brain (the hippocampus and amygdala) where partial seizures originate. While basic research could reveal stronger links between cannabinoids and seizure initiation, this does not seem as promising as other potential uses for marijuana-based medicines.

ALZHEIMER'S DISEASE

An estimated 4 million Americans currently have Alzheimer's dementia, a number that is likely to grow as the country's population ages. Alzheimer's is an incurable progressive disease of the nervous system that typically begins with memory loss and behavioral changes. At present, therapies for

Alzheimer's are limited to relieving its various symptoms. Even the two drugs, donepezil (Aricept) and tacrine (Cognex), that improve mental functions in some patients do not stop the progression of the disease.

There are two possible applications for cannabinoid treatments in Alzheimer's disease: to stimulate patients' appetites and to improve their behavior. Food refusal, which may be symptomatic of depression, is a common problem among people with Alzheimer's dementia; sometimes, but not always, antidepressant medications improve patients' appetites. Treatments would also be welcome that reduced agitation or antisocial behavior in Alzheimer's patients—behaviors that are not only unsafe but that also reduce caregivers' ability to help patients.

In one study, 11 Alzheimer's patients were treated with oral THC (dronabinol, Marinol) for six weeks, followed by six weeks of a placebo. Researchers found that the drug produced significant weight gain and reduced disturbed behavior without causing serious side effects.[10] Most of the patients were severely demented, and their memories were also seriously impaired. Although short-term memory loss is a common side effect of THC in healthy people, it was not measured in this study. In the future it would be useful to study how THC and other cannabinoids affect people with Alzheimer's whose memories remain largely intact. Such patients would be ill served by a medication that accelerated memory loss.

At the time of writing, additional clinical trials of Marinol in Alzheimer's patients and others with dementia appear likely to begin soon. In late 1998, Unimed Pharmaceuticals, which makes Marinol, received a U.S. patent for use of the drug in improving disturbed behavior in people with dementia, including the dementia of Alzheimer's and Parkinson's diseases.

NOTES

1. Consroe P, Sandyk R, Snider SR. 1986. "Open label evaluation of cannabidiol in dystonic movement disorders." *International Journal of Neuroscience* 30:277-282.

2. Richter A and Loscher W. 1994. "(+)-WIN55,212-2 a novel cannabinoid receptor agonist, exerts antidystonic effects in mutant dystonic hamsters." *European Journal of Pharmacology* 264:371-377.

3. Sandyk R, Consroe P, Stern P, Biklen D. 1988. "Preliminary trial of cannabidiol in Huntington's disease," in *Marijuana: An International Research Report*. Chesher G, Consroe P, Musty R, eds. Canberra, Australia: Australian Government Publishing Service.

4. Consroe P, Laguna J, Allender J, Snider S, Stern L, Sandyk R, Kennedy K, Schram K. 1991. "Controlled clinical trial of cannabidiol in Huntington's disease." *Pharmacology, Biochemistry, and Behavior (New York)* 40:701-708.

5. Frankel JP, Hughes A, Lees AJ, Stern GM. 1990. "Marijuana for Parkinsonian tremor." *Journal of Neurology, Neurosurgery, and Psychiatry* 53:436.

6. Hemming M and Yellowlees PM. 1993. "Effective treatment of Tourette's syndrome with marijuana." *Journal of Psychopharmacology* 7:389-391; Sandyk R, Awerbuch G. 1988. "Marijuana and Tourette's syndrome." *Journal of Clinical Psychopharmacology* 8:444-445.

7. British Medical Association. 1997. *Therapeutic Uses of Cannabis.* Amsterdam, The Netherlands: Harwood Academic Press.

8. Ng SKC, Brust JCM, Hauser WA, Susser M. 1990. "Illicit drug use and the risk of new-onset seizures." *American Journal of Epidemiology* 132:47-57.

9. Institute of Medicine. 1999. *Marijuana and Medicine: Assessing the Science Base.* Washington, DC: National Academy Press, pp. 170-172.

10. Volicer L, Stelly M, Morris J, McLaughlin J, Volicer BJ. 1997. "Effects of dronabinol on anorexia and disturbed behavior in patients with Alzheimer's disease." *International Journal of Geriatric Psychiatry* 12:913-919.

9

MARIJUANA AND GLAUCOMA

G laucoma ranks among the most frequently cited reasons for using medical marijuana and is one of the indications for which the federal government once granted permission for compassionate marijuana use (see Chapters 2 and 11). Research findings from as early as the 1970s show that both marijuana and THC reduce intraocular pressure, a key contributor to glaucoma. The first such reports generated considerable interest because at the time conventional medications for glaucoma caused a variety of adverse side effects. But, as will be described, other treatments for the disorder have since eclipsed marijuana-based medicines. Conventional therapies for intraocular pressure outperform cannabinoids, and the next generation of glaucoma drugs is expected to treat the disease more directly or even reverse its progress.

After cataracts, glaucoma is a leading cause of blindness worldwide, affecting more than 60 million people. Its most common form, primary open-angle glaucoma (POAG), is a slowly progressive disorder that destroys cells in the eye's retina and degrades the optic nerve. These losses constrict the visual field, which eventually disappears, along with the patient's sight.

Researchers have not yet learned what triggers POAG, but they have identified three factors that place individuals at risk for developing the disease: age, race, and elevated intraocular pres-

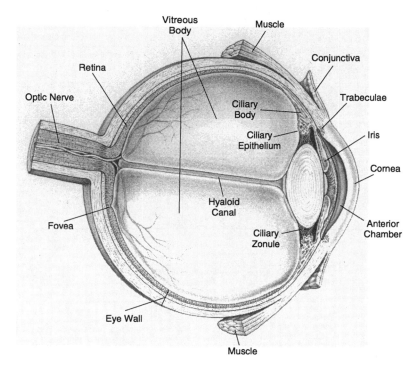

FIGURE 9.1 The anatomy of the human eye. (Drawing by Roberto Osti.)

sure. One percent of people age 60 have POAG, while more than 9 percent of people over 80 develop the disease. For African Americans the figure rises to 10 percent and is up to 25 percent among Caribbean people of African origin (who are less racially mixed than their American counterparts).

The third risk factor, elevated intraocular pressure, results from blockage in the flow of fluid that helps the eye maintain its rigid shape (see Figure 9.1). Normally this clear fluid, called the aqueous humor, circulates between the front of the lens and the back of the cornea. In people with elevated intraocular pressure the outflow of fluid from the anterior chamber of the eye becomes restricted, causing pressure to build up like water behind a dam. Increased pressure in the eye contributes to glaucoma by decreasing the flow of nutrients to the optic nerve, scientists suspect. Because elevated intraocular pressure is the only significant risk factor for glaucoma that can be controlled, most treatments to date have been designed to reduce it. Unfortunately, reducing intraocular pressure does not always stop or even slow the progress of glaucoma toward blindness.

Drugs can alter intraocular pressure by acting on different circulation routes of the aqueous humor (see Table 9.1). One important outflow route is the trabecular meshwork, a latticework of connective tissue and cells. The fluid flows through this tissue, into a little canal, and out of the eye, where it joins the bloodstream. Such drugs as epinephrine or dipevefrin work by chang-

TABLE 9.1 Treatments for Glaucoma

Drug class	Examples	How it reduces IOP
Beta-2 adrenergic agonists	epinephrine dipivefrin	Eases flow through trabecular meshwork
Beta-2 adrenergic antagonists	timolol betaxolol	Supresses production of aqueous fluid
Cholinergic agonists	pilocarpine	Eases flow through trabecular meshwork
Alpha-2 adrenergic agonists	aproclonidine brimonidine	Reduces production of aqueous fluid
Carbonic anhydrase inhibitors	acetazolamide dorzolamide	Reduces production of aqueous fluid
Prostaglandin-F_{2a} analogs	latanoprost unoprostone	Helps drain excess fluid

Surgery	How it reduces IOP
Laser modification of trabecular meshwork	Improves flow through meshwork
Drainage tube insertion	Helps drain excess fluid
Destruction of ciliary epithelium	Reduces fluid production

ing the shape of certain cells, resulting in improved flow through the trabecular meshwork. Pilocarpine, another type of drug, contracts the muscle that controls the shape of the trabecular meshwork making it easier for fluid to pass through, whereas timolol, yet another type of drug, interferes with fluid manufacture by the ciliary epithelium. Other drugs, such as apraclonidine and brimonidine, also reduce the amount of fluid produced. Finally, an additional type of drug simulates the production of agents that ease the passage of aqueous humor from the eye.

There are also surgical options for controlling elevated intraocular pressure. The trabecular meshwork can be cut with a laser, allowing the fluid to move out of it more easily. Alternatively, a surgeon can remove a piece of the eye wall and allow fluid to drain out under the conjunctiva. Doctors can also insert tiny drainage tubes, similar to those used for middle-ear problems, inside the eye to allow fluid drainage to the outer layers of the eye. Lastly, laser, heat, or cold can be used to destroy the ciliary epithelium, which secretes the aqueous humor.

Several clinical studies have found that cannabinoids or marijuana reduce intraocular pressure (IOP) as well as do most conventional glaucoma medications.[1] This is true whether the cannabinoids are administered orally, intravenously, or by inhalation but not when they are applied directly to the eye. Smoked or eaten marijuana, THC and synthetic cannabinoids in pill form, and intravenous injections of several natural cannabinoids have all been shown to reduce IOP significantly in both glaucoma patients and healthy adults with normal IOP. In most trials a single dose of marijuana or cannabinoid maintained this effect for three to four hours.

Researchers have yet to explain how marijuana and cannabinoids reduce IOP. But while clearly effective in reducing IOP, marijuana-based treatments for glaucoma have numerous drawbacks. Marijuana reduces blood pressure and produces psychological effects that some people—particularly the elderly—find intolerable. Several patients in these studies also reported that their hearts pounded or raced and that they felt uncomfortably anxious after taking cannabinoids. All of these effects could prove especially problematic for people at risk for cardiovascular disease and stroke; moreover, reduced blood pressure could decrease blood flow to the optic nerve, counteracting the benefits of reducing IOP. Finally, their short duration of effect means that marijuana-based medicines must be taken up to eight times a day, which most patients are unlikely to do; other medicines reduce IOP equally well and need only be taken once or twice a day. This is an important difference because patients need to control IOP continuously due to the progressive nature of glaucoma.

It is possible that future research could reveal a therapeutic effect for isolated cannabinoids other than THC or produce synthetic cannabinoid analogs that last longer and have fewer side effects. But the most promising line of research for treating glaucoma lies in the development of therapies that can protect or rescue the optic nerve from damage or that can restore its blood supply. There is some evidence that a synthetic cannabinoidlike compound known as HU-211 has nerve-protecting properties, although it does not reduce IOP. HU-211 is chemically similar to THC, but it is not found in the marijuana plant and does not bind to the cellular receptor in brain cells that THC activates.

There is no question that marijuana-based medicines can be used to lower IOP. But like several other glaucoma medications that have fallen into disuse, their drawbacks outweigh their benefits. This was not the case when the first reports of marijuana's effects on IOP were published in the 1970s, a time when relatively few drugs—all of which caused troubling side effects—were available to treat the condition. Those drugs have since been superseded by more effective and less problematic medications. That seems the likely fate of marijuana-based treatments for glaucoma as well.

NOTE

1. Institute of Medicine. 1999. *Marijuana and Medicine: Assessing the Science Base*. Washington, DC: National Academy Press, pp. 203-204.

III

MEDICAL MARIJUANA IN CONTEXT

P revious chapters reviewed what basic research and medical science have discovered so far about the medical use of marijuana. Cannabinoids—chemicals in marijuana and their synthetic relatives—were shown to affect a variety of physiological processes through their interactions with cellular receptors. The performance of marijuana and cannabinoids in clinical experiments designed to test their ability to relieve symptoms of several different disorders was also discussed.

The next three chapters place this knowledge in a broader context while considering the future of medical research on marijuana. Chapter 10 examines the economic realities of developing drugs based on active compounds from marijuana. Although most researchers who study cannabinoids would agree that the scientific route to cannabinoid drug development is clearly marked, there is no guarantee that the fruits of scientific research will be made available to the public. Marijuana-based medicines will become available only if there is enough financial incentive for the pharmaceuticals industry to invest in producing and marketing them or if public funding is available for research and development.

Meanwhile, despite the passage of several state referenda that support the medical use of marijuana, prescribing marijuana remains a federal offense. Marijuana is classified with heroin and LSD among federally controlled substances considered to have high potential for abuse and no accepted medical value. People suffering from debilitating symptoms that cannot be relieved with available drugs and who might find relief by smoking marijuana can take little comfort in a promise of a better cannabinoid drug 10 years from now. The health-related dangers of self-treatment with marijuana have already been addressed, but what about the legal consequences? Chapter 11 provides an overview of the current legal status of medical marijuana.

While legal issues related to medical marijuana have captured public attention in recent years, scientists have also demonstrated an increased interest in discovering and exploiting marijuana's medicinal benefits. After an initial burst of scientific activity in the 1970s, today's renewed interest grew out of several important discoveries made since 1986. These include the identification and cloning of human cannabinoid receptors, the discovery of natural compounds in the body that activate these receptors, and the creation of synthetic compounds that also activate cannabinoid receptors. Chapter 12 discusses the Institute of Medicine's recommendations—as well as those of other expert organizations—for building on these findings as we contemplate the future of marijuana-based medicine.

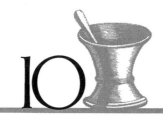

PHARMACEUTICALS FROM MARIJUANA

W hen the U.S. Food and Drug Administration approves the sale of a new medicine, its decision typically marks the conclusion of several years of expensive and labor-intensive development. Few compounds that appear promising in the early stages of research actually complete the journey from discovery to approval, and even fewer repay the cost of their development.

This is the path that novel medicines from marijuana compounds and their synthetic analogs must travel before reaching the pharmacy. But unless marijuana-based products can be made profitable as well as safe and effective, pharmaceutical firms are unlikely to pursue the research and development needed to produce them. This chapter examines the development of marijuana-based medicines from the perspective of their potential manufacturers. Along with the requirements for FDA approval, this chapter describes how the U.S. Drug Enforcement Administration (DEA) regulates marijuana and how marijuana's status as a controlled substance represents a potential barrier to developing cannabinoid medications.

Despite rather daunting odds, one cannabinoid product has been on the market for more than a decade: dronabinol, or synthetic THC. Currently sold as an oral medication under the brand name Marinol, dronabinol is being investigated for use in a variety of new applications. Its continuing story is recounted here—a story that offers insights into the development process—and a description of additional cannabinoids under development is provided. Finally, this chapter assesses the outlook for new marijuana-based drugs as well as prospects for marketing whole marijuana as medicine.

THE DRUG-APPROVAL PROCESS

Under the federal Food, Drug, and Cosmetic Act, the FDA decides whether a drug is sufficiently safe and effective to enter the marketplace. The agency bases its decision on evidence assembled from clinical trials conducted by the drug's sponsor. Pharmaceutical companies sponsor the majority of clinical trials, but academic and government laboratories also participate in drug development. For example, the National Institutes of Health funds collaborative programs to promote the commercial development of drugs for conditions such as AIDS, cancer, addiction, and epilepsy. Such programs supported most of the research that brought dronabinol to market.

Drug development begins with a compound that has either been synthesized in a chemical laboratory or purified from a natural source. If scientists find it has a useful biological activity, they will proceed to test the compound in animals in order to determine its effects on whole organisms. For example, after discovering that a compound extracted from a plant binds to receptors on nerve cells involved in appetite stimulation, researchers might perform tests to see if the compound could actually cause mice to increase their food consumption and gain weight. Such early experiments, which occur before human testing of an experimental medicine, are known as the preclinical phase of drug development.

When evidence from animal research suggests that a drug should be safe and effective in humans, the manufacturer submits an Investigational New Drug (IND) application to the FDA. The IND submission contains a plan for human clinical trials and documents the results of preclinical testing. If the FDA does not contest the IND within 30 days, the manufacturer may proceed to conduct clinical tests of the new drug in humans.

Clinical trials generally consist of three phases (see Figure 10.1). During Phase I, healthy volunteers take the drug to confirm that it is safe for human use and to determine dosage. In Phase II a small group of patients who have the condition intended for treatment with the experimental drug test the compound to evaluate its safety and its potential for causing side effects. If the drug passes the first two phases successfully, it proceeds to Phase III trials in larger groups of patients. These tests are designed to confirm that the drug is effective and to monitor any adverse reactions that might occur during long-term use.

Progress through all three phases takes an average of five years to complete, but a variety of factors can impede this process. Most important, researchers must be able to find enough volunteers to participate in trials; this is often difficult for the second and third phases since the pool of available patients may be small. In addition, several factors related to the specific compound can slow its passage through clinical trials. Generally, the more complex the experimental medicine or the disease or symptom being treated, the lengthier the clinical trial process. Drugs that produce multiple effects and those intended for long-term use— for example, to treat symptoms of chronic conditions such as AIDS or glaucoma—demand extra time in the clinic. But even a relatively straightforward passage through clinical testing consumes most of the $200 million to $600 million spent to develop the average drug.* And since only about one in five drugs that begin Phase I eventually secures FDA approval, clinical trials represent a significant financial risk.

Once a compound has passed all three phases of clinical testing, its manufacturer submits a request to market the drug, called a New Drug Application (NDA), to the FDA. An NDA is a massive document that includes not only the results of clinical testing but also of experiments designed to characterize the drug's chemistry and physiological activity as well as a detailed description of the process that will be used to manufacture it. In the case of a cannabinoid drug the NDA would probably also include the re-

---

* How best to estimate the cost of developing a drug is subject to debate. Different methods produce different estimates, but the general range is from $200 million to $600 million.

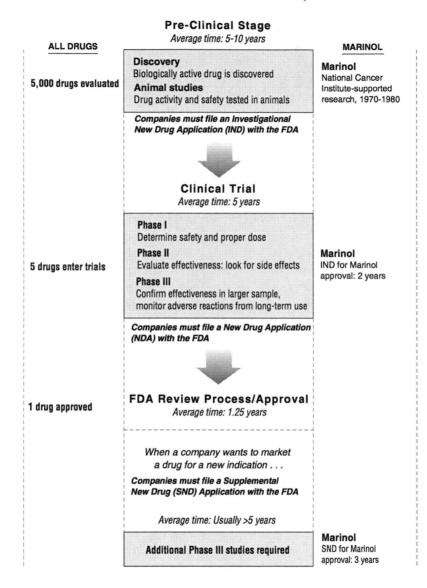

FIGURE 10.1 The drug development process consists of a series of stages. The process begins with the discovery of a biologically active drug and ends with the granting of approval for its sale by the Food and Drug Administration. Approximately one in five drugs that begin Phase I trials secure FDA approval.

sults of a series of studies designed to assess the drug's potential for abuse. In 1996 it took the FDA an average of 15 months to review and approve a successful NDA; in 1990 it took about two years. Federal legislation passed in 1992 that allowed the FDA to charge user fees to industry—and thereby hire additional reviewers—has greatly expedited this process.

The approval of an NDA by the FDA permits the drug's manufacturer to market it for the treatment of a single specific condition or symptom. Physicians are free to prescribe the drug for additional indications, a practice known as off-label use. To obtain permission to market an approved drug for additional indications, the manufacturer must submit a supplemental application to the FDA. This is usually a far simpler and less expensive process than the initial NDA, since the drug in question has already been proven safe and its side effects have been well characterized. Generally, the pharmaceutical company must conduct one or two new Phase III clinical studies to demonstrate an approved drug's efficacy in treating an additional indication, a process estimated to cost $10 million to $40 million.

Receiving FDA approval to market a drug for a new indication also takes time. Because the agency assigns lower priority to reviewing these so-called efficacy supplements than to evaluating NDAs, approval for a supplement has in some instances taken even longer than the original NDA. This process may eventually be reformed according to the Food and Drug Modernization Act of 1997, which allows manufacturers to provide information about off-label uses for drugs without prior FDA approval. However, since the new rules specified in this act are likely to be modified and refined in the courts, its ultimate impact remains uncertain.

Pharmaceutical companies must also get approval from the FDA before marketing an approved drug in a new dosage form. For example, if Unimed Pharmaceuticals, the manufacturer of Marinol, wanted to produce an inhaled version of the medicine, it would first have to conduct research to prove that the new delivery method is safe and effective. Moreover, in this particular case the company would probably also have to document the abuse potential of inhaled dronabinol.

While FDA approval represents a considerable hurdle in the

path toward developing novel cannabinoid drugs, the agency also sponsors two programs that may encourage progress in this area. One program, authorized under the Orphan Drug Act of 1983, provides incentives to manufacturers to develop drugs to treat rare so-called orphan disorders. Such diseases, by definition, affect no more than 200,000 people in the United States. Since drug companies are unlikely to recoup the costs of developing medicines for so few patients, the FDA offers a variety of economic incentives that allow firms to make a profit from orphan drugs, including the right to an exclusive market for their product for seven years. Some of the medical conditions for which cannabinoids show promise, such as spasticity or Huntington's disease, may meet the definition of an orphan disease.

In addition, disorders affecting more than 200,000 people in the United States may contain subgroups that qualify as orphan populations. For example, while Parkinson's disease affects approximately 1 million Americans, a small number of these patients may share a specific symptom, such as early-morning motor dysfunction, that can be relieved by an orphan drug. The FDA can also grant orphan drug privileges to a medicine intended for more than 200,000 patients if it will cost more to develop than the manufacturer can recover in profits.

The second FDA program that might expedite cannabinoid drug development is known as the treatment IND. It allows patients with life-threatening diseases, such as AIDS or cancer, access to experimental medications before they have received approval for marketing. Once a drug enters Phase III clinical trials, treatment INDs may be issued to allow patients who are not part of the trials to use the drug as long as no comparable approved medication exists. This program might thus permit some patients to try a promising novel cannabinoid much sooner than if it followed standard FDA procedure. Success at this early stage could boost sales of the drug once it was approved for widespread marketing.

SCHEDULING OF CONTROLLED SUBSTANCES

The federal Controlled Substances Act of 1970 requires that every drug with a potential for abuse, including marijuana and compounds derived from it, be classified and regulated according to whether there is a currently accepted medical use for the drug as well as the likelihood that the drug will be abused. The DEA conducts the classification process, assigning each controlled substance into one of five categories called schedules (see Box 10.1). Each schedule invokes a specific set of regulatory controls on research, manufacturing, distribution, prescription, sale, and use of the drug. For example, patients who take morphine, a Schedule II medication, must appear in person to have their prescriptions filled, rather than phone in their requests to the pharmacy.

The possibility that a drug might be scheduled under the Controlled Substances Act represents a major deterrent to its development by a pharmaceutical company because scheduling can limit its profits in two main ways. First, the company must document the drug's abuse potential, which adds to research costs as well as the time it takes to bring the drug to market. Testing for abuse liability may require the manufacturer to conduct studies on both animals and humans to gauge the likelihood that people will want take the drug for nonmedical purposes. These studies attempt to predict whether the drug might be sold on the black market or otherwise pose a threat to public health. The second drawback of scheduling for pharmaceutical companies is the tendency of physicians to avoid prescribing scheduled drugs, which further reduces potential sales.

The scheduling of a controlled substance may be initiated by any of several parties, including the DEA, the U.S. Department of Health and Human Services (DHHS), the drug's manufacturer, or by public petition. Final rulings on scheduling rest with the DEA, in consultation with the secretary of the DHHS, who makes his or her recommendation (which the DEA usually follows) after reviewing the relevant scientific evidence. Once the DEA receives a DHHS scheduling recommendation for a particular drug, it usually takes weeks to months for the agency to announce its decision. In addition to scheduling at the federal level by the DEA, several states also impose scheduling laws of their own on the manufacture and distribution of controlled substances.

Currently, tetrahydrocannabinols, including THC and all other chemically related compounds derived from the marijuana

Box 10.1
Scheduling Definitions for Controlled Substances as
Established by the Controlled Substances Act of 1970

Schedule I (includes heroin, LSD, and marijuana)
    (A) The drug or other substance has a high potential for abuse.
    (B) The drug or other substance has no currently accepted medical use in treatment in the United States.
    (C) There is a lack of accepted safety for the use of the drug or other substance under medical supervision.

Schedule II (includes methadone, morphine, methamphetamine, and cocaine)
    (A) The drug or other substance has a high potential for abuse.
    (B) The drug or other substance has a currently accepted medical use in treatment in the United States or a currently accepted medical use with severe restrictions.
    (C) Abuse of the drug or other substances may lead to severe psychological or physical dependence.

Schedule III (includes Marinol, anabolic steroids)
    (A) The drug or other substance has a potential for abuse less than the drugs or other substances in Schedules I and II.

plant, are assigned to the most restrictive category (Schedule I) because they have no currently accepted medical use and have a high potential for abuse. Synthetic cannabinoids with activity similar to THC would also be automatically assigned to Schedule I, according to DEA regulations. An exception to this is dronabinol (Marinol); initially a Schedule II drug, it was reassigned to Schedule III in July 1999 as a result of a petition filed by its manufacturer.

Both the FDA and the DEA tightly regulate research on Schedule I substances, even when it does not involve human trials. For example, scientists studying cannabinoids found in marijuana plants must first receive DEA approval of both their experimental plans and their research facilities (see Chapter 11). Because com-

(B) The drug or other substance has a currently accepted medical use in treatment in the United States.

(C) Abuse of the drug or other substance may lead to moderate or low physical dependence or high psychological dependence.

Schedule IV (includes Valium and other tranquilizers)

(A) The drug or other substance has a low potential for abuse relative to the drugs or other substances in Schedule III.

(B) The drug or other substance has a currently accepted medical use in treatment in the United States.

(C) Abuse of the drug or other substance may lead to limited physical dependence or psychological dependence relative to the drugs or other substances in Schedule III.

Schedule V (includes codeine-containing analgesics)

(A) The drug or other substance has a low potential for abuse relative to the drugs or other substances in Schedule IV.

(B) The drug or other substance has a currently accepted medical use in treatment in the United States.

(C) Abuse of the drug or other substance may lead to limited physical dependence or psychological dependence relative to the drugs or other substances in Schedule IV.

SOURCES: 21 U.S.C. §812 and 21 C.F.R. 1308, April 1, 2000.

pliance with these regulations is both costly and time consuming, few pharmaceutical companies are likely to undertake such studies. By contrast, cannabinoids that are not found in the marijuana plant and that are chemically distinct from THC, including anandamide and several synthetic cannabinoids currently being evaluated in preclinical studies, were not classified as controlled substances at the time of writing. These compounds therefore represent more attractive candidates for drug development than their marijuana-derived counterparts. Nevertheless, since a cannabinoid from a source other than marijuana has yet to be tested in clinical trials in the United States, it remains to be seen whether such compounds will continue to remain unscheduled.

It is too soon to tell to what extent scheduling will affect the overall development of cannabinoid drugs. On an individual basis, cannabinoids are likely to be scheduled if they exist naturally in the marijuana plant, if their chemical structure or pharmacological activity resembles that of THC, or if they otherwise show potential for abuse. If a cannabinoid is actually derived from marijuana, it automatically falls under Schedule I. To market such a cannabinoid as a medicine, the manufacturer would first have to petition the DEA to have it rescheduled—a strong disincentive to developing such drugs.

Of course, the rescheduling of marijuana to a less restrictive category would drastically change the outlook for cannabinoid drug development. The National Organization for the Reform of Marijuana Laws (NORML) and others continue to petition the DEA to remove marijuana and THC from Schedule I; so far these efforts have been unsuccessful. If marijuana were to be rescheduled, that decision would result in the rescheduling of any cannabinoid found in the plant.

THE MARINOL STORY

Marinol is the brand name for an oral form of dronabinol, the only marijuana-based prescription medicine currently available in the United States. Each gelatin-coated Marinol capsule contains 2.5, 5, or 10 milligrams of dronabinol—a synthetic compound identical to natural THC—dissolved in sesame oil. The only difference between THC and dronabinol is their origins. Both are the products of a series of chemical reactions; those that produce THC occur in plants, while those that produce dronabinol take place in a laboratory or chemical factory. Rather than perform an expensive extraction to purify THC from marijuana plants, which are illegal to grow in the United States, Unimed Pharmaceuticals manufactures Marinol from pure dronabinol.

To date, Marinol has received FDA approval for two applications: to control nausea and vomiting associated with cancer chemotherapy and to counteract AIDS wasting. However, as will be discussed later in this section, dronabinol appears promising for additional indications and may also be adaptable to several new delivery methods, so it is likely to be marketed more widely in the future. Another synthetic cannabinoid, nabilone (Cesamet), has been approved for use in the United Kingdom. A close relative of THC, nabilone is also prescribed for chemotherapy-induced nausea and vomiting.

Dronabinol's greasy consistency presents several problems to a drug manufacturer. First, it makes the compound difficult and expensive to purify. Second, because dronabinol does not dissolve readily in water, only a fraction of the orally ingested compound reaches the patient's circulation. That amount is further reduced by the action of the liver, which recognizes dronabinol as a contaminant and removes it from the bloodstream. As a result, researchers have estimated that only 10 to 20 percent of the dronabinol in each capsule actually reaches its target in the body: cells bearing cannabinoid receptors (see Chapter 2).

Compared with other oral medications, dronabinol takes effect quite slowly. Absorption through the gastrointestinal tract is inherently slow; however, a typical over-the-counter pain reliever achieves results within 30 minutes, while dronabinol's peak activity does not occur until two to four hours after ingestion. This is not the case when dronabinol is injected or inhaled. Delivered by these methods, the drug reaches its maximum level in the body nearly instantaneously because it enters the bloodstream immediately (inhaled dronabinol is absorbed directly into capillaries in the lungs). While peak dronabinol concentrations may vary greatly among patients who take it orally, inhalation and injection produce more consistent levels of the drug.

Another drawback of dronabinol use is the frequency of side effects, most of which involve the nervous system. These include anxiety, confusion, dizziness, mood changes, sleepiness, and thinking abnormalities. In two recent clinical trials about one-third of patients who received dronabinol reported having such symptoms, although only a small number of these patients actually discontinued their use of the drug.[1] Reducing the dose of dronabinol appears to minimize most of its adverse side effects, particularly feelings of disquiet or malaise.

Given the considerable challenges of bringing Marinol to market, it may seem remarkable that Unimed accomplished that task. But the company had plenty of help in the form of government-sponsored research on THC and incentives for drug development. Most of the preclinical and clinical studies on THC that culminated in the initial FDA approval of Marinol in 1985 were conducted or funded by the National Cancer Institute beginning in the 1970s. Unimed estimates that it contributed only about one-quarter of the total research effort that secured Marinol's entry into the U.S. market. Its development also proceeded more quickly than usual, moving from IND to approval in two years, compared with five years for the average drug.

Unimed later applied for FDA approval to market Marinol for a second indication—AIDS wasting. At that time, the agency required Unimed to complete two relatively small Phase III studies, which lasted three years and cost approximately $5 million—again, a relative bargain in terms of both time and money. Under the Orphan Drug Act, the FDA also granted Marinol seven years of exclusive marketing for this application, beginning with its approval in 1992.

After Marinol received FDA approval for AIDS wasting in 1992, its sales grew significantly. This gain was especially welcome, since profits from medication for chemotherapy-induced nausea were beginning to decline as a result of the introduction of more effective antinausea drugs, such as ondansetron, that are also unscheduled.

Since its commercial introduction in 1985, Marinol had been listed in the most restrictive schedule for medically useful controlled substances along with morphine, cocaine, and other prescription medications with a "high potential for abuse." While such a distinction clearly limited Marinol's availability, it did not delay the drug's initial entry into the market because the scheduling decision was made by the DEA prior to FDA approval; nor did any delays occur as a result of state scheduling laws.

When Unimed later prepared to petition the DEA to reschedule Marinol, the company commissioned a study to determine the extent to which its product was being abused. The study was conducted by researchers at the Haight Ashbury Free Clinic in San Francisco—where significant numbers of marijuana users, as well as people with HIV and AIDS, receive treatment—and it included information gathered from addiction medicine specialists, oncologists, cancer and AIDS researchers, and law enforcement officials.[2] The researchers reported that they found no evidence that Marinol was being abused or diverted from medical use.

They attributed the drug's low abuse potential to the fact that it is slow to take effect and also because of the negative mood changes it sometimes produces.

In July 1999 the DEA granted Unimed's petition to reschedule Marinol from Schedule II to Schedule III. This action lifted many of the restrictions that previously limited Marinol's availability. Now physicians who prescribe Marinol in quantity or who specify refills face far less cumbersome paperwork than when the drug was listed in Schedule II. Not surprisingly, Unimed estimates that moving Marinol to Schedule III could produce a 15 to 20 percent increase in the drug's sales, currently estimated at $20 million (a modest figure by industry standards).

Beyond this important gain, Marinol's market could expand even further if the drug were approved for additional indications. Currently, 80 percent of the patients using Marinol take it to relieve AIDS wasting, 10 percent to relieve chemotherapy-induced nausea, and the remaining population for off-label conditions. The latter group is thought to consist mainly of Alzheimer's patients; in a recent study the drug showed promise in treating appetite loss and behavioral disturbances associated with that disease. Unimed cannot, however, market Marinol to treat complications of Alzheimer's disease without first receiving FDA approval.

The company is currently conducting research in pursuit of approval for this indication and in late 1998 received a use patent for the application of Marinol to improve disturbed behavior in people with various forms of dementia, including Alzheimer's disease. This gives Unimed 20 years of patent protection for dementia treatments based on its product provided that the additional indication gains FDA approval.

Another likely market for Marinol consists of people with AIDS who receive combination antiretroviral therapy (see Chapter 5). For these patients dronabinol offers a double benefit: not only does the drug stimulate appetite, it also appears to relieve nausea and vomiting, common side effects of the standard daily doses of antiretroviral drugs. Unimed is presently conducting a Phase II study in this area; if the results are promising, the company plans to seek FDA approval for the additional indication.

In addition to possible applications for Alzheimer's and AIDS patients, Unimed—along with its marketing partner, Roxane

Laboratories—is exploring the possibility of using dronabinol to treat spasticity in multiple sclerosis as well as intractable pain. The companies are also studying its ability to stimulate appetite in people with cancer and renal disease. Each group of patients would represent a significant new market for the drug.

While expanding the number of approved indications for dronabinol represents an important route to increasing its sales, making a more effective version of the drug could potentially give it an even bigger boost. As described earlier, dronabinol is slowly and poorly absorbed. It is also difficult to find the right dose for each patient because it takes several hours for the drug's effects to reach their peak. Moreover, as with any oral drug, much of the initial dose is lost due to inefficient absorption or is destroyed in the liver. Thus, it makes sense that Unimed and Roxane are also pursuing new ways to deliver dronabinol that would avoid these pitfalls.

In 1998 Unimed filed an IND as a step toward developing four new formulations for dronabinol designed to deliver the drug more rapidly to the bloodstream. These include an inhaler, a method the IOM researchers consider to be particularly promising, and two nasal preparations, a spray and a gel. The company is also exploring oral formulations that would allow dronabinol to be absorbed directly into the blood vessels that lie beneath the tongue, rather than swallowed as a pill.

Other researchers are exploring the use of rectal suppositories to deliver THC or dronabinol, but this method is considerably slower than the previous four; it is also likely to be acceptable to fewer patients. Unfortunately, attempts to deliver THC through the skin, via a transdermal patches like those used to deliver nicotine or hormone therapy, have so far been unsuccessful. However, if chemists were to find a way to synthesize a THC analog that penetrated the skin more effectively, it could be delivered this way.

While more efficient methods of administering dronabinol, particularly the inhaled aerosol and spray routes, promise more rapid relief from symptoms that respond to the cannabinoid, they also carry an increased potential for abuse. As addiction experts have observed, the more rapidly a drug takes effect, the more likely it is to be abused. Unimed anticipates that FDA approval of more efficient delivery methods may require the company to determine their liability for abuse as well as their efficacy and physiological characteristics. Unimed estimates that each new formulation will cost between $7 million and $10 million to develop.

These additional research costs are likely to affect the price of new dronabinol formulations. In capsule form, dronabinol (Marinol) currently costs about $200 per month for its most common use—to combat AIDS wasting; the cost of treating chemotherapy-induced nausea is lower, since it is not a chronic condition. Several patients who spoke at the IOM's public workshops found Marinol's price to be prohibitive and said that one of the advantages of using marijuana for medical purposes was its relatively low cost. But this is a deceptive comparison, for the indirect costs of marijuana use—criminal penalties (see Chapter 11)—can be prohibitive. Moreover, marijuana users assume the risks of using a substance of uncertain quality and composition.

In fact, it is almost impossible to directly compare the costs of Marinol and medical marijuana use. The cost of Marinol varies, depending on the patient's situation. Public and private health insurance plans generally reimburse for all or part of the cost of Marinol but not, of course, for marijuana. Roxane Laboratories also sponsors an assistance program to provide Marinol for indigent patients. The price of marijuana is also quite variable; at California buyers' clubs, the IOM team learned, patients typically paid $2 to $16 per gram, depending on the grade of marijuana. (An average marijuana cigarette weighs approximately 1 gram.) Street prices are even less consistent, as is the quality of the product. The THC concentration of marijuana can easily vary from 2 to 15 percent. And while home cultivators can produce quality marijuana at low cost they also bear an increased risk of criminal penalty.

Based on the above considerations, Unimed has estimated that Marinol is in fact cheaper than marijuana for patients with health insurance or for those eligible for financial assistance from Roxane. For those who must assume the entire cost of Marinol out of pocket, it may still be cheaper than using whole marijuana if the patient smokes two or more average-sized joints per day. If medical marijuana were to become legally available, these comparisons would no longer hold. But for the moment Unimed believes that only a small portion of its potential market for Marinol is being lost to competition with marijuana.

While Marinol embodies the promise of cannabinoid medicines for treating multiple indications through a variety of delivery methods, its history also reflects the numerous challenges involved in developing such products. From purification and delivery, to the costs of research and regulatory compliance, to the difficulties of marketing a controlled substance, the barriers to producing cannabinoid drugs are many. It is also important to remember that government support for the research and development of Marinol significantly lowered these hurdles. Thus, while instructive, the exact conditions that produced Marinol are unlikely to be duplicated for another cannabinoid drug.

Turning from this specific case, we now examine the factors that are likely to determine whether new medicines will continue to be developed from marijuana, the outlook for drugs based on individual cannabinoid compounds, and the prospects for developing medicines from the entire marijuana plant.

PROSPECTS FOR NOVEL CANNABINOID MEDICATIONS

The potential therapeutic value of cannabinoids extends far beyond remedies for nausea and weight loss. As detailed in previous chapters, marijuana and THC have already shown some promise in treating pain and muscle spasms and in providing simultaneous relief for several symptoms, particularly in AIDS patients. Although all of these conditions represent opportunities to fulfill unmet patient needs, pharmaceutical companies must weigh additional factors in determining whether to pursue the development of marijuana-based therapies.

Before assuming the financial risk of initiating preclinical research or clinical trials, manufacturers must first determine whether such investments are likely to produce adequate returns. These decisions are typically made on the basis of a market analysis, an attempt to forecast the potential costs and benefits of developing a specific drug. For cannabinoid drugs, the development costs will probably be higher than average because of the additional expense of testing for abuse liability. And if the compound under consideration is classified as either a neuropharmaceutical or a nonsteroidal antiinflammatory drug—the two therapeutic categories associated with the highest development costs—the price of approval could rise even higher.

To estimate potential returns from a candidate drug, a pharmaceutical company assesses several contributing factors. It calculates the drug's projected market size based on the estimated patient population, sales of existing medications, and the degree to which existing drugs will compete with a new product. The company would also consider whether patients will use the drug for a limited time or whether it will be used to treat chronic condition. Treatments for chronic conditions that emerge early in life are especially valuable from a commercial standpoint.

The ability to patent a candidate drug also affects its potential market since it gives the holder the exclusive right to sell a novel and non-obvious product for 20 years. Other types of market protections, such as orphan drug status, confer similar advantages. As discussed earlier, scheduling under the Controlled Substances Act tends to decrease the market for a drug, as do adverse side effects and interactions with other medications. Finally, markets may be swayed by other less predictable factors, such as social attitudes—an important consideration for marijuana-based medicines—and the likelihood that insurers will reimburse patient costs.

Several companies and individuals have presumably weighed these factors and decided in favor of pursuing cannabinoid drugs since the public record shows that at least three such compounds are currently being developed (see Table 10.1). According to the IOM, all of these compounds, except dronabinol (THC) and marijuana, remain in the preclinical stage.

The list of cannabinoids in Table 10.1 is far from comprehensive. Other firms may be working on related compounds and keeping their progress a secret; since IND information is confidential, it is even possible that clinical trials on additional cannabinoids are under way. Researchers have also produced a wide variety of natural and synthetic cannabinoids for experimental purposes that may have therapeutic applications. In addition, uses may be found for cannabinoids that are currently suspended or withdrawn from pharmaceutical development.

Based on the information in Table 10.1, we can draw three

TABLE 10.1 Cannabinoids Under Development for Human Use as of July 2000

Name of Drug	Possible Indication(s)	Investigator	Stage of Development	FDA Status
HU-211 (Dexanabinol)	Neuroprotection (Neurotrauma, stroke, multiple sclerosis, Parkinson's, Alzheimer's)	Pharmos Corp.	Phase II trial completed March 2000 in Israel; Contract for Phase III trial awarded June 2000	None
CT-3	Antiinflammatory Analgesia	Atlantic Pharmaceuticals	Phase I trial in France	IND
THC (Marinol)	[see text]	Unimed Roxane Labs	Phase I trials in U.S.	IND
Marijuana Plant	Multiple sclerosis, spinal cord injury, pain	GW Pharmaceuticals	Phase I trial completed in England; Phase II trial begun May 2000	None
	HIV-related appetite stimulation	Donald Abrams, University of California at San Francisco	Phase I trial completed May 2000	IND

Source: Adapted from Institute of Medicine. 1999. *Marijuana and Medicine: Assessing the Science Base*. Washington, DC: National Academy Press, p. 209.

tentative conclusions about the present state of cannabinoid drug development. First, nearly all of the investigators listed are either small companies or individuals, who are generally willing to assume greater commercial risk than a large pharmaceutical company. Because such small enterprises typically obtain funding from venture capital, stock offerings, or collaborations with larger companies rather than from sales, they can pursue riskier goals.

Second, except for THC and marijuana, no plant-derived cannabinoids appear in Table 10.1. While a number of such compounds have shown promising results in animal and human experiments (see Chapter 2), commercial interest in them appears to be lacking. This is probably due to several factors. First, under the Controlled Substances Act, such compounds would initially be placed in Schedule I; even if the necessary rescheduling proceeded smoothly, controlled substances carry a stigma that limits their sales potential. An additional deterrent to developing cannabinoids from the marijuana plant is the fact that such natural products are ineligible for product patents. Plant-derived compounds may, however, secure use patents such as those awarded to dronabinol and other orphan drugs. Finally, chemical analogs of plant-derived compounds, which could be patented, may offer improved solubility, fewer side effects, or benefits over their natural counterparts.

The third point apparent from Table 10.1 is that cannabinoids are being considered for even more applications than were discussed in previous chapters. One of the most prominent among these additional uses is neuroprotection, which involves rescuing nerve cells from destruction due to trauma, oxygen deprivation, or neurological disease. Cannabinoids are thought to provide this protection through their association with receptors on nerve cells (see Chapter 2). Also, both THC and cannabidiol can act as potent antioxidants to protect nerves from toxic forms of oxygen that arise when the body is under stress.

Another antioxidant, the synthetic cannabinoid HU-211, also has been shown to protect nerve cells from exposure to excessive amounts of the neurotransmitter glutamate, a byproduct of trauma or disease. The cannabinoid acts by blocking glutamate receptors on the neuron, thereby preventing glutamate and other damaging agents from binding.[3] HU-211 has been tested for safety in humans in the United Kingdom and has progressed to Phase II clinical trials in Israel for the treatment of severe brain injury.[4]

In addition to these possibilities, several plausible scenarios might encourage pharmaceutical firms to pursue marijuana-based products in the future. If cannabinoids seemed likely to fulfill important unmet medical needs, their development might be worth the financial risk. Pain relief represents such a potential market; in 1997 Americans spent an estimated $4.4 billion on prescription and over-the-counter pain relievers. Yet there is a long-standing need for medicines to treat both acute and chronic pain that are safe, nonhabit forming, and easy for patients to take. A cannabinoid medication with these attributes would be a welcome addition to existing therapies.

Another group of potentially lucrative compounds act by binding cannabinoid receptors without activating them, thereby producing the opposite effect of molecules that activate the receptor. Similar effects also could be achieved with compounds that interfere with receptor binding by natural cannabinoids. Neither class of drugs would be subject to the same scheduling restrictions as natural cannabinoids or their mimics because abuse of such products is unlikely. And since such compounds are not derived from marijuana, both types of drugs could receive product patents. Similarly, one could envision another related class of compounds capable of increasing the synthesis of natural cannabinoids or interfering with their breakdown. Such drugs would probably be scheduled, though, because they could increase the concentration of cannabinoids in the body, creating conditions that might produce the marijuana "high" and therefore the potential for abuse.

Scientists have already synthesized several chemicals that affect interactions between cannabinoids and their cellular receptors. To date, these compounds have largely been used as tools to probe cannabinoid function, but they produce physiological effects of their own and may thus prove therapeutically useful. For example, since THC reduces short-term memory, a drug that prevents THC from binding cannabinoid receptors might enhance memory. Similar blockers might prevent cannabinoid-induced immune suppression (see Chapters 2 and 3), while drugs that exert the opposite effects of THC, thereby suppressing the appetite, could potentially promote weight loss.

As marijuana-based medicines currently under development proceed through the regulatory pipeline, pharmaceutical firms will be watching. If this handful of experimental drugs perform well in the clinic, receive FDA approval with relative ease, avoid scheduling restrictions, and above all turn a profit, more companies are likely to pursue similar compounds. Since industry experience to date is limited to the case of Marinol, and most of its developmental costs were borne by the U.S. government, it remains to be seen whether other cannabinoid drugs can survive the rigors of development. For the present, both the apparent dearth of compounds and the small size of the companies involved attest to the high risk of such a venture.

PROSPECTS FOR MEDICAL MARIJUANA USE

The possibility that marijuana itself will emerge as a new medicine is far more remote than the prospects for drugs based on individual chemicals derived from the plant. Along with many of the downside risks associated with the approval and scheduling of cannabinoid drugs, medicinal marijuana faces several additional barriers to development. Thus, it is not surprising that FDA approval has never been sought for the medical use of marijuana.

The first hurdle presents itself early in the development process: conducting research on marijuana. As discussed in greater detail in the next chapter, obtaining research-grade marijuana and the legal permission to study it are difficult and time-consuming endeavors. At present the only existing IND for medical marijuana authorizes a Phase I (safety) study on the treatment of AIDS wasting with smoked marijuana.

Before marijuana could be marketed legally in the United States, it would have to satisfy a long list of regulatory requirements. As a botanical product, marijuana could, in theory, be classified as dietary supplement. Most herbal medicines fall into this category, which exempts them from FDA review. But since marijuana is also a controlled substance, it is unlikely that it would ever win approval for sale without restriction and probably not without obtaining FDA approval in the form of an NDA.

While the FDA is currently developing standards to review botanicals as drugs, no such preparation on the market today has received the agency's approval. Indeed, appraising whole-plant medicines is problematic since it is difficult to assure that such products will remain consistently stable, potent, and free of contamination over time. A medical marijuana preparation would, presumably, need to meet all of these standards. An even greater obstacle to development lies in the fact that marijuana is smoked, which represents a significant safety risk (see Chapter 2). Marijuana delivered by a vaporizing device that permits inhalation of cannabinoids while filtering out carcinogens would still require

FDA approval but would allay many smoking-related safety concerns.

Moreover, marijuana could only be brought to market if it were rescheduled to acknowledge its "accepted medical use," according to DEA standards. To meet that requirement, a compound must have a known and reproducible chemical structure; its safety and efficacy must be proven; its use must be approved by qualified experts; and scientific evidence for its medical use must be widely accepted. Yet even if all of these criteria were satisfied and marijuana were rescheduled, international treaties may prevent it from being classified in a less restrictive category than Schedule II.

Finally, because marijuana is a natural product, it cannot be patented under U.S. law. Only new marijuana strains not found in nature might be eligible for a product patent, which prohibits anyone else from selling an identical strain for 20 years. A Dutch company, HortaPharm B.V., has developed several unique marijuana strains and has registered them in Europe but has not yet applied for a patent in this country. In fact, marijuana from HortaPharm cannot presently enter the United States because Dutch authorities have refused to issue the necessary export permit (the DEA has approved the importation of HortaPharm plants for research purposes, however).

The path to developing the whole marijuana plant as a medication is so crowded with scientific, regulatory, and commercial roadblocks that it seems highly unlikely to be taken. The appearance of new cannabinoid pharmaceuticals, while more promising, is still years away. Meanwhile, patients, caregivers, policymakers, and voters are weighing the legal consequences of using marijuana for medical purposes. The next chapter explores the legal landscape surrounding the medical use of marijuana, which both influences and is influenced by scientific knowledge of the drug's effects.

Notes

1. Beal JE, Olson RLL, Morales JO, Bellman P, Yangco B, Lefkowitz L, Plasse TF, Shepard KV. 1995. "Dronabinol as a treatment of aneorexia associ-

ated with weight loss in patients with AIDS." *Journal of Pain and Symptom Management* 10:89-97; Beal, JE, Olson R, Lefkowitz L, Laubenstein L, Bellman P, Yangco B, Morales JO, Murphy R, Powderly W, Plasse TF, Mosdell KW, Shepard KV. 1997. "Long-term efficacy and safety of dronabinol for acquired immunodeficiency syndrome-associated anorexia." *Journal of Pain and Symptom Management* 14:7-14.

2. Calhoun SR, Galloway GP, Smith DE. 1998. "Abuse potential of dronabinol (Marinol)." *Journal of Psychoactive Drugs* 10(2):187-196.

3. Shohami E, Weidenfeld J, Ovadia H, Vogel Z, Hanus L, Fride E, Breuer A, Ben-Shabat S, Sheskin T, Mechoulam R. 1996. "Endogenous and synthetic cannabinoids: Recent advances." *CNS Drug Reviews* 2:429-451; Striem S, Bar-Joseph A, Berkovitch Y, Biegon A. 1997. "Interaction of dexanabinol (HU-211), a novel NMDA receptor antagonist, with the dopaminergic system." *European Journal of Pharmacology* 388:205-213.

4. Knoller N, Levi L, Israel Z, Razon N, Reichental E, Rappaport Z, Ehrenfreund N, Fiegon A. 1998. "Safety and outcome in a Phase II clinical trial of dexanabinol in severe head trauma." Congress of Neurological Surgeons Annual Meeting, Seattle, October 7.

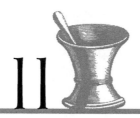

LEGAL ISSUES

Although the focus of this book—and of the IOM report on which it is based—is on science, such knowledge does not exist in a vacuum. The scientific evidence of marijuana's potential risks and benefits as a source of medicine needs to be considered in a social context. That is true whether the decision at hand concerns the care of a single patient or the law of the land.

Much has been written about the impact of marijuana laws on society, a topic that often overshadows science in debates concerning marijuana's worth as a medicine. We will not attempt to address this complex subject, nor do we provide anything remotely resembling legal advice, which should be sought from a professional. The aim here is simpler: to give an overview of marijuana's legal status as both a medicine and a source of new pharmaceuticals. The previous chapter described how economic issues affect marijuana-based drug development; this chapter explores the influence of the law on medical use of marijuana.

Because marijuana legislation has changed markedly over the past 70 years and will probably continue to do so, our survey is at best a snapshot of a moving target. This is particularly true at the state level, where laws vary widely; local enforcement is even more variable. The picture is considerably clearer at the national level, and it applies to every resident of the United States (except for a handful of isolated cases, which we will subsequently describe): to use marijuana, even if solely to relieve medical symptoms, is to violate federal law. This fact should be kept in mind in reading this chapter.

Readers should also note that, while much of this chapter concerns the medicinal use of smoked marijuana, it is not intended as an endorsement of this practice. Rather, it is a reflection of the primitive stage of development of marijuana-based therapeutics—that is, compared with modern expectations that drugs should be proven effective before they are prescribed. Since cannabinoid medications other than Marinol or a smoke-free vaporizer are probably years away, the issue of marijuana's legal status is bound to concern today's patients at least as much as its promise as a source of new medicines.

FROM MEDICINE TO ILLICIT DRUG

Long before marijuana acquired its reputation as a substance of abuse, it was regarded as a folk medicine in several cultures. In the United States, patent remedies contained extracts of the marijuana plant well into the 1930s; by that time, though, doctors were far more likely to prescribe opiates or synthetic drugs such as barbiturates for conditions once treated with marijuana. Then, for three decades after passage of the federal Marijuana Tax Act in 1937, the drug essentially disappeared from medical use in this country.[1]

Several states had already outlawed marijuana for nonmedical purposes by 1920. These laws were passed mainly in reaction to reports of marijuana use among Mexican immigrants, who introduced the drug to the United States. Congress later drafted the Marijuana Tax Act in an attempt to quash the spread of marijuana use without interfering with the rights of individual states to regulate drug sales.

Although the tax act allowed medical use of marijuana, it created a formidable bureaucracy with which few doctors or pharmaceutical firms were willing to contend. Manufacturers and medical users of the drug were required to comply with burdensome registration procedures and pay a tax of $1 per ounce. By contrast, marijuana for nonmedical use—the act's intended target—was taxed at the prohibitive rate of $100 per ounce. In 1942 marijuana lost its legitimacy as a prescription medication when it was removed from the *United States Pharmacopoeia (USP).*

Few Americans were familiar with marijuana in the late 1930s and even fewer had tried the drug. Its use was limited almost entirely to Mexican immigrants, except in a handful of cities where artists, students, and musicians experimented with it. As a result, there was little dissent when the federal government sought to tax marijuana out of existence. The only exception was the American Medical Association (AMA), whose objections to the Marijuana Tax Act were twofold: that scientific data on marijuana's harmful effects were lacking and that the act would impede investigation of potential medical uses of the drug.[2] As Congress considered passage of the law, the AMA's legislative activities committee wrote in protest:

> Cannabis at the present time is slightly used for medicinal purposes, but it would seem worthwhile to maintain its status as a medical agent.... There is [also] the possibility that a restudy of the drug by modern means may show other advantages to be derived from its medicinal use.[3]

The Marijuana Tax Act successfully curtailed marijuana's spread until the 1960s, when recreational use of the drug surged far beyond previous levels. In response to this development and also out of an effort to consolidate and reform federal narcotics laws, Congress passed the Comprehensive Drug Abuse Prevention and Control Act in October 1970. The portion of this law that concerns drug classification and control, known as the Controlled Substances Act (CSA), has remained largely unchanged since its inception. According to the CSA, drugs with potential for abuse are placed into one of five categories called schedules. The assignment of a drug to a particular schedule is supposed to take into account the likelihood that it will cause physical and psychological dependence, as well as its medical utility (see Box 10.1). The lower the schedule number of a given drug, the higher an abuse risk it presents, and the greater the restrictions on access to it. For example, LSD and heroin appear in Schedule I, along with marijuana; Schedule V lists pain relievers that contain codeine.

Efforts to reschedule marijuana commenced with passage of the CSA. In 1972 NORML filed a petition with the federal government, which was denied two years later. NORML continued to press for public hearings on the issue, which were finally held between 1986 and 1988. Once again, however, the DEA rejected NORML's position and that of several additional supporting groups, despite recommendations to the contrary by the administrative law judge in charge of the case.[4] The rescheduling advocates then petitioned for a review of the case by the U.S. Court of Appeals, which eventually denied the request in February 1994.[5]

In contrast to these unsuccessful attempts to reschedule marijuana, its principal psychoactive ingredient, THC—in the form of the prescription drug dronabinol (Marinol)—has twice been rescheduled and is now listed in Schedule III. After receiving FDA approval in 1985, the drug was moved from Schedule I to Schedule II, enabling physicians to prescribe it. In July 1999 dronabinol was once again rescheduled following a petition from Unimed Pharmaceuticals, the company that manufactures Marinol. The drug is now listed in a category reserved for substances, such as anabolic steroids, that can produce low-to-moderate physical dependence or high psychological dependence.

A MEDICAL NECESSITY?

With the rise in marijuana use in the 1960s, a few Americans discovered its medicinal properties either through contact with cultures where it was used as a folk remedy or simply by noting that their symptoms improved after smoking marijuana. Among them was Robert Randall, a glaucoma patient whose troubles led to two important legal developments concerning medical marijuana use: the creation of a government-sponsored marijuana treatment program and the birth of the "medical necessity" defense against the charge of marijuana possession.

In 1975 Randall was arrested for cultivating marijuana on his porch in Washington, D.C. He admitted that the plants were his but claimed that he grew them to treat the symptoms of glaucoma and thereby preserve his eyesight. At the time of his arrest, Randall's vision was already greatly impaired; conventional drugs, which initially controlled the damaging pressure in his eyes, had ceased to help him. He won the ensuing case, *Randall v. United States*, on the grounds that marijuana use kept him from becoming blind. The federal government then looked for a way to provide other such patients with marijuana.

A solution to this dilemma, the Compassionate Use Program, was launched in 1976. It was administered as part of an existing program to provide seriously ill patients with promising medicines prior to their approval by the FDA. Thirteen patients were accepted into this program between 1976 and 1991. They received government-grown marijuana to treat a variety of symptoms and were later joined by hundreds of patients in state-run experimental treatment programs. To obtain this legal marijuana, a patient's physician—or the physician in charge of the state program—submitted a lengthy application to the FDA, after which the DEA conducted inspections to assure that the drug would not be diverted from its intended use. Then, as now, the National Institute on Drug Abuse (NIDA)—an arm of the National Institutes of Health—oversaw the cultivation and distribution of all marijuana provided by the U.S. government.[6]

In 1991 the Public Health Service closed the Compassionate Use program for smoked marijuana after a National Institutes of Health review concluded that marijuana was not the best treatment for any of the patients who were receiving it. Increasing numbers of AIDS patients were applying to the program, and its administrators worried that smoking marijuana would be harmful to people with compromised immune systems. At the time the program closed, 28 people had been approved for treatment, but only the 13 who were already receiving marijuana continued to have it provided to them. Since then five of those original patients have died of AIDS. Most state-sponsored clinical research programs folded in the 1980s due to lack of patient interest and after 1986 due to their inability to obtain research-grade marijuana from the federal government.

Upon reconsidering the Compassionate Use suspension in 1994, the Clinton administration decided to keep the program closed. However, with the recent release of the IOM report to the White House's Office of National Drug Control Policy, the subject of government-sponsored marijuana use has again come under federal scrutiny.

Rather than argue for the resurrection of the suspended program, the IOM team advocated support for research that could further the development of a smoke-free cannabinoid delivery system. The team also wrote: "We acknowledge that [at the present time] there is no clear alternative for people suffering from conditions that might be relieved by smoking marijuana." Such patients could be treated as the subjects of individual clinical trials that would be overseen by a medical review board. Patients would receive marijuana to smoke under close medical supervision and only after being informed of their status as experimental subjects using a harmful drug delivery system. The results of these studies would increase scientific understanding of the risks and benefits of marijuana use, the IOM researchers contended.

The IOM researchers recommended pursuing two types of short-term (less than six months) clinical trials of smoked marijuana: for conditions that appear likely to be improved with such treatment and for patients with debilitating, otherwise incurable symptoms such as chronic pain or AIDS wasting. They did not recommend such trials to promote the smoking of marijuana but rather because such trials could help accelerate the development of a smoke-free cannabinoid delivery system.

While the Compassionate Use program for marijuana smokers now exists solely as a historical artifact, the medical necessity defense remains viable for some patients who treat their symptoms with marijuana. This defense originates from the common law principle that illegal actions are excusable or justified if they are taken to avoid even greater harms. Courts considering such cases must balance the interest of the individual patient against the government's interest in upholding the law.

The specific requirements to mount a defense of medical necessity for marijuana use vary from state to state. In most cases, patients must show that they used marijuana in order to avoid serious medical harm. To do so, the defense typically calls the treating physician or another medical expert to testify that marijuana relieves the patient's symptoms. The defense must also convince the judge or jury that the harm of breaking the law in question is less severe than the harm the patient would suffer if deprived of marijuana. Many courts also require patients to prove that no legal alternative treatment exists; this is often a major point of contention between the prosecution and defense in medical marijuana cases.[7]

Legal experts regard the medical necessity defense as an extremely demanding one and note that it fails as often as it succeeds.[8] Among the more frequently cited successes is the case of Samuel Diana, a multiple sclerosis patient convicted of marijuana possession in the state of Washington. In appealing Diana's conviction the defense relied on testimony from physicians and other people with MS as well as from Diana himself. The court concluded that marijuana minimized Diana's symptoms, that no other drug would be as effective, and that the benefits of his marijuana use outweighed the harm to society of his criminal action. The court also emphasized that its decision applied only to Diana and his specific circumstances.[9]

In a similar case tried in Idaho in 1990 (*State v. Hastings*) the court refused to establish a specific defense of medical necessity in a case of marijuana possession. Nonetheless, it did entitle the defendant, who had rheumatoid arthritis, to employ a more general defense of necessity as stated in common law. Once this defense was allowed, the prosecutor dropped all charges against the defendant.[10]

The medical necessity defense also has failed for a variety of reasons. Some defendants have lost because they did not make an effort—futile though it might have been—to obtain marijuana through legal channels such as the federal Compassionate Use or state research programs. Others have aroused the skepticism of the judge or jury by growing or possessing exceptionally large amounts of marijuana. In one case (*Commonwealth v. Hutchins*), tried in Massachusetts in 1991, the court refused to acknowledge the existence of a medical necessity defense. Dissent from this decision led the state to establish a marijuana research law and the governor to pardon the defendant.[11]

The advent of new cannabinoid drugs or delivery systems that could replace smoking for some patients may eventually restrict the applicability of the medical necessity defense. On the other hand, the discovery of new medicinal applications for marijuana could result in its expansion. Either way, medical marijuana users should bear in mind that this already unreliable tactic continues to be subject to change.

Even more important, patients should understand that the medical necessity defense has not been recognized by courts or legislatures in most parts of the country. Further, under current federal law there is no legal means to obtain marijuana for medical use. Violators of federal law risk prosecution, imprisonment, fines, and forfeiture of property. State laws concerning medicinal marijuana use and possession, discussed in the next section, vary widely in terms of penalties.

MEDICAL MARIJUANA AND THE STATES' LAWS

While marijuana is regulated at the federal level as a substance without medicinal value, laws in several states recognize and make allowances for a variety of therapeutic uses. This situation presents a troubling paradox for patients, caregivers, and physicians: if they use, procure, or recommend marijuana for medical purposes in compliance with state law, they are guilty of a federal crime.

State laws permitting the medical use of marijuana vary widely and apply to a broader range of situations than individual necessity cases. However, most state laws on medical marijuana belong to one of three general categories. First, several states created therapeutic research programs to study marijuana's effects on seriously or terminally ill patients. Some states have granted permission to physicians to recommend marijuana for such patients. Lastly, some states have established their own controlled substances regulations in which marijuana has been assigned to Schedule II (a largely symbolic measure since the federal CSA prevails).[12] Two groups that advocate legalizing medical marijuana, NORML and the Marijuana Policy Project, maintain databases of state marijuana laws on their web sites.

Since state marijuana laws can not be implemented without cooperation from the federal government, medical marijuana laws enacted in more than 20 states have had little practical effect. This is particularly true where the state stipulates that marijuana for medical purposes must be obtained through a clinical research program, since these programs no longer exist, except on paper. Several factors contributed to the demise of state-sponsored clinical programs, including the federal government's refusal to provide them with marijuana after 1986.

Lack of patient interest also helped doom these programs,

most of which focused on relieving chemotherapy-induced nausea. Many of the mostly older participants in such trials dropped out after having adverse reactions to smoked marijuana (see Chapter 6). Other patients and their physicians were discouraged from participating by the burdensome paperwork involved. The fate of several moribund state programs was then sealed with the 1985 approval of dronabinol (Marinol), which led state boards of health to conclude that marijuana was obsolete as a medicine. As a result, by the time the spread of AIDS produced a new group of patients seeking help from marijuana, neither state nor federal Compassionate Use programs were available to them.

The demands of these patients, along with a general increase in marijuana's medicinal properties, led voters in California to pass a state medical marijuana initiative in 1996. Known as Proposition 215, it permits patients and their primary caregivers, with a physician's recommendation, to possess and cultivate marijuana for the treatment of AIDS, cancer, muscular spasticity, migraines, and several other disorders; it also protects them from punishment if they recommend marijuana to their patients. Since 1996, voters in five other states—Alaska, Arizona, Nevada, Oregon, and Washington as well as the District of Columbia—have approved similar measures, all in direct conflict with federal law. (Although exit polls indicated that voters in the District of Columbia approved the measure by a 69 percent majority, Congress refused to allow the ballots to be counted and nullified the referendum.)

Time has shown, however, that medical marijuana initiatives are much easier to pass than they are to implement. As long as marijuana remains in the federal government's Schedule I, the threat of prosecution to anyone involved with its procurement or use has deterred all but a minority of doctors, patients, and providers of medical marijuana from establishing public distribution contemplated by the new state laws.[13]

For physicians the potential consequences of recommending marijuana to patients include the loss of DEA licenses to prescribe controlled substances as well as cancellation of Medicare and Medicaid contracts. These were among the threats made by federal officials to California doctors following passage of Proposition 215, and they have apparently served to deter many physicians—including those in other states—from recommending marijuana to their patients or even discussing it with them.

Physicians remain wary despite a temporary injunction issued by U.S. District Judge Fern Smith in April 1997 preventing the federal government from restricting doctors' right to discuss marijuana with their patients. Such discussions, the judge ruled, are protected as free speech under the First Amendment. Nevertheless, the distinction between recommending marijuana use and "aiding and abetting" patients in obtaining an illicit substance is a fine one, as several state medical associations have noted. For example, in a 1999 bulletin entitled "Medical Use of Marijuana," the Washington State Medical Association cautions its members as follows:

> Physicians must not prescribe marijuana. It is prohibited under federal law to knowingly or intentionally distribute, dispense, or possess marijuana. The terms "distribute" and "dispense" have been widely interpreted, and physicians may be found in violation of federal law for writing a prescription for a substance, such as marijuana, for which federal law has no recognized medical use. Violation of federal law can bring significant penalties, including imprisonment and fines. In addition, violating federal law (or aiding and abetting in its violation) may result in other physician sanctions, such as a revocation of a physician's DEA registration.

The bulletin advises doctors who recommend marijuana to provide a signed statement, or a copy of the patient's medical records, indicating "that in the physician's professional opinion, the potential benefits of marijuana outweigh the risks" for the individual.

Of course, patients who use marijuana as a medicine also risk criminal conviction. Even where recent voter initiatives exempt such use from state criminal penalties, it is still subject to federal prosecution. As a result, most people who turn to marijuana to relieve their symptoms do so in secrecy and without the full knowledge or consent of a doctor. Most medical users get their marijuana through the same means as recreational users: from friends who give or sell it to them, by growing it themselves, or by buying it "on the street" from professional dealers.

A minority of medical users—perhaps 10 percent, according to Chuck Thomas of the Marijuana Policy Project—make use of so-called cannabis buyers' clubs. Most visible in California, buyers' clubs originated with AIDS patients who initially formed the groups to distribute herbal medicines and imported pharmaceuticals not approved for sale in the United States. When club members found that marijuana relieved some of their symptoms, they organized supply networks, which eventually expanded to include people with other disorders.

Most buyers' clubs continue to be small and secretive; some are barely distinguishable from the informal relationships that form between many medical marijuana users, growers, and dealers. But in California, as well as such cities as New York, Seattle, Key West, Washington D.C., and Portland, Oregon, several larger buyers' clubs have begun to operate openly in recent years. Ensuing state and federal lawsuits have forced many of these public clubs to close. Those that remain open do so in cooperation with local authorities. Others have been replaced by more "low-key" distribution networks.

There is no such thing as a typical buyers' club. Each has its own culture, determined to a large extent by its policies, patients, and physical location (see Figure 11.1). Some clubs act as marijuana purchasing agents, others as cooperative associations of patients and sometimes growers. Patients can smoke or eat marijuana on the premises at a few clubs, but most tend to operate like pharmacies, dispensing a variety of types and grades of marijuana, often at or below cost. Clubs generally require patients to present some kind of medical documentation, such as a physician's referral, in order to receive marijuana.

At the time of writing, the future of public buyers' clubs appears to be uncertain, largely as a result of a series of lawsuits brought by the federal government against six of the most visible California clubs in 1998. The suits, which remain in litigation, can be viewed as a test of the federal government's ability to enforce the CSA in states that have enacted medical marijuana initiatives.

In at least one case, local governments have attempted to protect buyers' clubs from federal interference. When the Oakland Cannabis Buyers' Cooperative was targeted for closure in 1998, the city responded by designating its employees as officers of the city (ironically, by granting them the same privileges as undercover narcotics agents). This tactic failed to save the club, how-

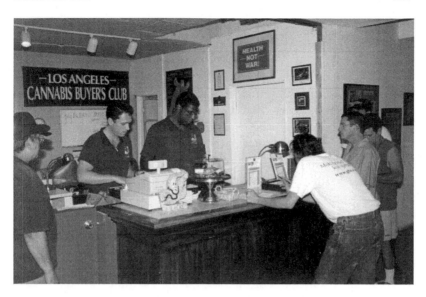

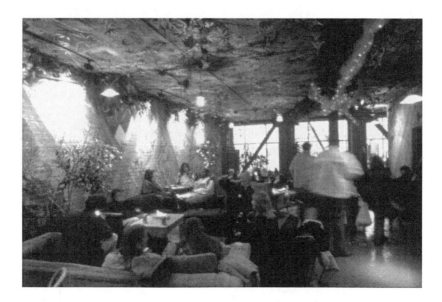

FIGURE 11.1 Contrasting photos of cannabis buyers' clubs in Los Angeles and San Francisco, California. (Top photo by Tyler Hubby, Los Angeles Cannabis Resource Center, identifiable people: Jay Fritz, Mirron Willis, Craig Poore, and Michael Goldberg. Bottom photo by André Grossman, San Francisco Buyer's Club.)

ever. Bowing to federal pressure, the cooperative ceased marijuana and at the time this book was written, operated only as a patient registration center. But in July 2000, a ruling of the Federal District Court restored the right of the Oakland club to distribute marijuana to patients with a serious medical condition who will suffer imminent harm without marijuana, and who have no legal alternative to marijuana for effective treatment for their illness. It is unclear how many of the club's members meet these criteria, but the ruling at least admits the possibility that the Oakland club, as well as others in California, could reopen.[14]

The federal government also succeeded in closing perhaps the most notorious of all buyers' clubs: the San Francisco Cannabis Cultivators' Club. In this case, however, local authorities acted to support, rather than thwart, the federal government's efforts. Unlike the Oakland cooperative, which resembled a pharmacy, the San Francisco club not only allowed smoking on the premises but encouraged members to do so by providing them with comfortable lounges and a "cannabis bar." Registration procedures were reportedly lax, and little effort was made to confirm members' claims of medical need. Several less flamboyant Bay Area buyers' clubs now serve former members of the San Francisco club.

At the opposite end of the cannabis club spectrum, the Los Angeles Cannabis Resource Center remains untouched by federal lawsuit. Open since November 1996, the LACRC dispenses marijuana for home consumption only. The club also offers legal assistance, volunteer programs, and support groups for members and their caregivers, who must be at least 18 years old. Nearly 80 percent of the center's more than 650 active members are AIDS patients.

To receive marijuana, patients are required to submit a statement signed by a licensed California physician stating that he or she recommends or approves use of the drug. A staff member then calls the physician to verify this information, which is updated annually. To ensure the quality of the marijuana it dispenses, the LACRC obtains 70 percent of its supply from a garden on the premises and from other co-op members who grow marijuana at home. The remainder is acquired from independent growers.

No one is more aware of the precarious legal position held by the LACRC than its director, Scott Imler. But Imler, an architect of Proposition 215, sees buyers' clubs as an interim solution to the medical marijuana problem. Like most of the patients he serves, he would prefer marijuana to be prescribed and dispensed by a pharmacist, as an FDA-approved medication. Unless and until that happens, the relative safety and low-cost products offered by buyers' clubs—whether public or underground—are likely to continue to attract a significant minority of medical marijuana users.

RESEARCH AND REGULATION

One point on which both sides in the medical marijuana debate can agree is the need for definitive clinical research on marijuana. As a National Institutes of Health committee noted in 1997, "until studies are done using scientifically acceptable clinical trial design and are subjected to appropriate statistical analysis, the questions concerning the therapeutic utility of marijuana will likely remain much as they have to date—largely unanswered."[15]

But in order to conduct such research, scientists must thread their way through a complex maze of regulations, beginning with the restrictions imposed by the federal Controlled Substances Act. To use a Schedule I substance such as marijuana in a clinical study, researchers must first be judged qualified and competent by the DHHS, which must also approve the study plan. The applicants may then proceed to the DEA to receive a special registration that allows them to use marijuana for research purposes. In addition, some states have their own controlled-substances laws, adding another regulatory layer. Moreover, studies designed to test marijuana's therapeutic properties must also receive approval from the FDA (see Chapter 10).

Beyond obtaining all necessary federal and state approvals as well as funding for their study, scientists proposing to conduct research on marijuana must procure an adequate supply of the drug. Researchers cannot simply grow the marijuana they need but instead must acquire it from the federal government, according to international law. As a party to the United Nations Single Convention on Narcotic Drugs, the United States has agreed to establish a national agency to cultivate and distribute marijuana for scientific and medical purposes. Currently, that responsibility rests with NIDA; NIDA also screens all research projects for which it provides marijuana.

NIDA grows its marijuana on a Mississippi farm. A North Carolina factory processes some of the crop into cigarettes, available in a range of THC concentrations, as well as a placebo. Until recently, NIDA provided this marijuana free of charge, but only for use in studies funded by the National Institutes of Health. Revised procedures issued in May 1999 make it available to researchers supported by other governmental agencies or private organizations.[16] But all researchers, except for those funded by NIDA itself, must now reimburse the agency for the cost of raising, processing, and distributing the marijuana they use.

While NIDA's revised policies may encourage more studies of marijuana's potential medical benefits, they also impose clear limits on the nature of such research. Guided by the Institute of Medicine's report as well as the findings of the National Institutes of Health's expert panel, NIDA announced that it would give priority to studies on the development of alternative delivery systems for marijuana or its constituent cannabinoids. The agency also stated that it would favor research on patients with serious or life-threatening conditions or those for whom no therapies exist.

Much to the dismay of medical marijuana advocates, NIDA did not announce the return of a compassionate use program or even support for ongoing trials of medical marijuana. Instead, NIDA guidelines state that preference will be given to multipatient studies with specific endpoints. Rather than develop whole marijuana as a licensed drug, the stated goal of the NIDA program is to determine whether active compounds in marijuana can be safely delivered as medications that meet the FDA's standards for pharmaceuticals. These policies follow the recommendations stated in the IOM report, which emphasized that even trials of smoked marijuana be directed toward developing smokeless delivery systems for cannabinoids.

In August 1999, Health Canada—the equivalent of the DHHS—announced its support for a program of medical research on marijuana with aims similar to those stated in the NIDA guidelines. The Canadian agency will provide research-grade marijuana for approved studies and up to $1.5 million a year in funding through 2004. Studies of smoked marijuana will receive support only if they use the drug to treat terminally ill patients or are used in short-term clinical trials as a basis of comparison with other therapies. As in the United States, researchers must submit an IND application to the Canadian equivalent of the FDA before beginning clinical trials.

Health Canada's advisory committee declined to specify particular symptoms as acceptable candidates for experimental treatment with marijuana. By contrast, the NIDA guidelines refer applicants to recommendations made by the 1997 National Institutes of Health Workshop on the Medical Utility of Marijuana. That panel identified several promising therapeutic areas for marijuana research, including neuropathic pain, muscular spasticity, glaucoma, and wasting syndromes of AIDS and cancer.

The workshop report also notes the heavy regulatory burden on researchers who study controlled substances, particularly Schedule I substances such as marijuana. As a result, the report concludes, many scientists "have been discouraged from pursuing research with these substances." A 1995 IOM report on the development of addiction medication reached much the same conclusion, leading its authors to recommend that federal regulations be modified to remove barriers to research on controlled substances.[17]

NIDA's new guidelines may make marijuana more widely available for clinical studies, but they also leave intact regulations that pose significant hurdles to marijuana research. Whether the promise of marijuana-based medicines will lure scientists to overcome these barriers remains to be seen, but at the moment such a change appears unlikely. At the time of this writing, nearly nine months after NIDA published its revised guidelines, the agency had received only two requests for research-grade marijuana.

NOTES

1. Bonnie RJ and Whitebread CH. 1974. *The Marihuana Conviction: A History of Marihuana Prohibition in the United States.* Charlottesville: University

Press of Virginia; Aldrich M. 1997. "History of therapeutic cannabis," in *Cannabis in Medical Practice*, Mathre ML, ed. Jefferson, NC: MacFarland and Co.

2. *Report of the Council of Scientific Affairs.* 1997. Report to the American Medical Association House of Delegates. Subject: Medical Marijuana. Chicago: AMA.

3. Grinspoon L. 1971. *Marihuana Reconsidered.* Cambridge, MA: Harvard University Press.

4. Drug Enforcement Agency. Marijuana Rescheduling Petition, Docket No. 86-22, Opinion and Recommended Ruling, Findings of Fact, Conclusions of Law and Decision of Administrative Law Judge Francis L. Young, September 6, 1988.

5. *Alliance for Cannabis Therapeutics v. DEA*, No. 92-1168, No. 92-1179, 15 F.3d 1131, U.S. Court of Appeals for the District of Columbia Circuit (1994).

6. Zeese K. 1997. "Legal issues related to the use of medical marijuana," in *Cannabis in Medical Practice*, Mathre ML, ed. Jefferson, NC: MacFarland and Co.; National Organization for the Reform of Marijuana Laws (NORML). Website visited July 22, 1999.

7. Kent NE. 1997. "People behind the pain," in *Cannabis in Medical Practice*, Mathre ML, ed. Jefferson, NC: MacFarland and Co.

8. NORML website.

9. Ibid.; Dogwill N. 1998. "The burning question: How will the United States deal with the medical-marijuana debate?" *Detroit College of Law at Michigan State University Law Review*, Spring.

10. Kent NE. 1997.

11. Ibid.; Dogwill N. 1998.

12. Kent NE. 1997.

13. Goldstein E. In preparation. "Implementation of Medical Marijuana Referenda: A Study of California, Washington, and Oregon." Unpublished paper.

14. Ruling in California Favors the Medicinal Use of Marijuana. *New York Times.* COL 02, P 17. Tuesday July 18 2000

15. National Institutes of Health. 1997. Workshop on the Medical Utility of Marijuana. *Report to the Director, National Institutes of Health, by the Ad Hoc Group of Experts.* Bethesda, MD: National Institutes of Health.

16. National Institutes of Health. 1999. Announcement of the Department of Health and Human Services' Guidance on Procedure for the Provision of Marijuana for Medical Research.

17. Institute of Medicine. 1995. *The Development of Medications for the Treatment of Opiate and Cocaine Addictions: Issues for the Government and Private Sector.* Washington, DC: National Academy Press.

12

Marijuana's Medical Future

W hile much of the IOM team's efforts focused on reviewing the accumulated scientific evidence of marijuana's medical risks and benefits, the team also charted a course for future research. With this goal in mind, the authors of the IOM report issued six recommendations regarding the continued study and use of marijuana and cannabinoids for medicinal purposes. This chapter discusses those proposals in detail, compares the conclusions of the IOM report with several other recent reports on medical marijuana, and considers the implications of the IOM team's findings for the future of marijuana-based medicine.

The IOM Recommendations

A complete list of the study team's recommendations, exactly as they appear in *Marijuana and Medicine: Assessing the Science Base,* is shown in Box 12.1. Appropriately, the first of these recommendations supports the continuation of basic studies to learn more about how the active ingredients in marijuana affect the body. Over the past two decades research in this area has begun to demonstrate how THC and related natural and synthetic cannabinoids exert their effects on individual cells. Scientists have also discovered that the human body produces substances that

Box 12.1
IOM Recommendations on Marijuana and Medicine

RECOMMENDATION 1: Research should continue into the physiological effects of synthetic and plant-derived cannabinoids and the natural function of cannabinoids found in the body. Because different cannabinoids appear to have different effects, cannabinoid research should include, but not be restricted to, effects attributable to THC alone.

Scientific data indicate the potential therapeutic value of cannabinoid drugs for pain relief, control of nausea and vomiting, and appetite stimulation. This value would be enhanced by a rapid onset of drug effect.

RECOMMENDATION 2: Clinical trials of cannabinoid drugs for symptom management should be conducted with the goal of developing rapid-onset, reliable, and safe delivery systems.

The psychological effects of cannabinoids are probably important determinants of their potential therapeutic value. They can influence symptoms indirectly which could create false impressions of the drug effect or be beneficial as a form of adjunctive therapy.

RECOMMENDATION 3: Psychological effects of cannabinoids such as anxiety reduction and sedation, which can influence medical benefits, should be evaluated in clinical trials.

Numerous studies suggest that marijuana smoke is an important risk factor in the development of respiratory diseases, but the data that could conclusively establish or refute this suspected link have not been collected.

RECOMMENDATION 4: Studies to define the individual health risks of smoking marijuana should be conducted, particularly among populations in which marijuana use is prevalent.

Because marijuana is a crude THC delivery system that also

delivers harmful substances, smoked marijuana should generally not be recommended for medical use. Nonetheless, marijuana is widely used by certain patient groups, which raises both safety and efficacy issues.

RECOMMENDATION 5: Clinical trials of marijuana use for medical purposes should be conducted under the following limited circumstances: trials should involve only short-term marijuana use (less than six months), should be conducted in patients with conditions for which there is reasonable expectation of efficacy, should be approved by institutional review boards, and should collect data about efficacy.

If there is any future for marijuana as a medicine, it lies in its isolated components, the cannabinoids and their synthetic derivatives. Isolated cannabinoids will provide more reliable effects than crude plant mixtures. Therefore, the purpose of clinical trials of smoked marijuana would not be to develop marijuana as a licensed drug but rather to serve as a first step toward the development of nonsmoked rapid-onset cannabinoid delivery systems.

RECOMMENDATION 6: Short-term use of smoked marijuana (less than six months) for patients with debilitating symptoms (such as intractable pain or vomiting) must meet the following conditions:

• failure of all approved medications to provide relief has been documented,
• the symptoms can reasonably be expected to be relieved by rapid-onset cannabinoid drugs,
• such treatment is administered under medical supervision in a manner that allows for assessment of treatment effectiveness, and
• involves an oversight strategy comparable to an institutional review board process that could provide guidance within 24 hours of a submission by a physician to provide marijuana to a patient for a specified use.

act on cannabinoid receptors and that this "cannabinoid system" appears to influence movement, memory, immunity, and pain sensation (see Chapter 2). The more research reveals about the diverse effects of various cannabinoids, the greater the likelihood that scientists will develop cannabinoid drugs that effectively treat specific symptoms, with a minimum of adverse side effects.

The second recommendation encourages the development and clinical testing of cannabinoid medicines for a few promising indications: pain relief, control of nausea and vomiting, and appetite stimulation. It also emphasizes the need to develop safer and more effective methods for administering these drugs to patients. While smoking marijuana allows cannabinoids to take effect rapidly and permits patients to titrate their dose—that is, to inhale just enough to achieve relief from their symptoms—it also has numerous drawbacks, particularly for people with health problems (see Chapter 3). Oral THC (in the form of dronabinol, sold as Marinol) has received approval from the FDA for treatment of nausea and vomiting as well as appetite loss. But Marinol takes effect slowly and cannot be effectively titrated by the user. Vomiting, in particular, would be far more amenable to treatment by inhalation than with a pill that needs to stay down.

The IOM team also urged, in its third recommendation, that clinical trials be designed to gauge the psychological effects of cannabinoid drugs. Marijuana's active ingredients, especially THC, produce feelings of well-being, calm, and sedation in many people. These effects could augment other therapeutic benefits of cannabinoids for some patients, but others may mistake good feelings for relief from their symptoms. The more researchers learn about how cannabinoids' physical and psychological effects interact, the better they can put the compounds to medical use.

Marijuana smoking clearly harms the cells of the respiratory system, in much the same way tobacco smoke does. But since no definitive study has shown that smoking marijuana causes cancer or chronic obstructive pulmonary disease, the IOM team called for such research in its fourth recommendation. Many studies suggest that marijuana smoke plays a role in causing respiratory disease, but no firm evidence exists to either support or refute this conclusion. This question is particularly important to AIDS patients who smoke marijuana to soothe several symptoms of their chronic disease and to combat adverse side effects of life-saving medications. Although the authors of the IOM report did not generally endorse the medical use of smoked marijuana, they concluded that its safety should be studied because significant numbers of patients use it to medicate themselves.

The IOM team also recommended pursuing clinical trials to determine how well smoked marijuana relieves certain medical symptoms. Such studies, the report suggests, should be conducted only under extremely limited circumstances and should be subject to review and approval by a board of experts. Patients with symptoms that are likely to be relieved by smoking marijuana would do so for six months or less, and their response to treatment would be recorded. Such experiments would not be directed toward establishing crude smoked marijuana as a conventional treatment but with the goal of assisting the development of a rapid smokeless method for administering pure cannabinoids.

The IOM team's final recommendation concerns short-term use of smoked marijuana by individual patients to relieve such symptoms as debilitating pain or nausea that have defied all conventional treatments. Physicians would present a scientifically and ethically based protocol for a single patient clinical trial to a regulatory board and apply for permission to prescribe marijuana to such patients on an experimental basis. In light of patients' acute discomfort, the board should provide a quick response—within 24 hours of a doctor's request. Physicians would not only supervise patients' use of the drug but would also collect data on how effectively it relieved their symptoms.

OTHER REPORTS ON MARIJUANA AS MEDICINE

During the three years preceding publication of the IOM's study on marijuana and medicine, several important reports on the same subject were released by other panels of scientific and medical experts. A summary of some of their conclusions, along with those of the IOM report, appears in Table 12.1. Readers should bear in mind that each of these reports was written for a different purpose, so it is difficult to make many direct comparisons. Nevertheless, all reached the same general conclusions: that marijuana can be moderately effective in treating a variety of

TABLE 12.1 Conclusions[1]

Report	Conditions recommended for treatment in clinical trials of smoked marijuana	Promising targets for cannabinoid drugs
Institute of Medicine[2]	Various, including nausea and vomiting, wasting, pain	Various, including nausea and vomiting, wasting, pain
House of Lords (U.K.)[3]	Multiple sclerosis, chronic pain	Not discussed
World Health Organization[4]	Not discussed	Nausea and vomiting; muscle spasticity
National Institutes of Health[5] (U.S.)	Wasting, chemotherapy-induced nausea and vomiting, neurological and movement disorders, glaucoma	Nausea and vomiting, neuropathy, possibly muscle spasticity, certain dystonias and epilepsy
British Medical Association[6]	Not discussed	Muscle spasticity, neurodegenerative disorders, epilepsy
American Medical Association[7]	Various, including AIDS, wasting, chemotherapy-induced nausea and vomiting, MS, spinal cord injury, neuropathy	Not discussed

[1]Institute of Medicine. 1999. *Marijuana and Medicine: Assessing the Science Base.* pp. 244-255.

[2]Institute of Medicine 1999.

[3]House of Lords (United Kingdom Parliament). Science and Technology Committee 9th Report. *Cannabis: The Scientific and Medical Evidence.* London: Her Majesty's Stationery Office.

[4]World Health Organization. 1997. Cannabis: a health perspective and research agenda.

Recommended research on potential harms of marijuana and cannabinoids?	Use of whole and/or smoked marijuana as medicine	Primary goals of cannabinoid drug development
Yes, especially on smoking-related harms	Whole marijuana is not a modern medicine	Safe, reliable, rapid-onset delivery method for cannabinoids
None recommended	Hazards of marijuana smoke noted	Rapid-onset, smoke-free delivery systems (e.g., inhalation, under the tongue, and rectal suppositories)
Various, including infertility, respiratory damage, immune dysfunction, schizophrenia, and "amotivational syndrome"	Hazards of marijuana smoke noted	Not discussed
None recommended	Should be held to same standards of safety and efficacy as other FDA-approved drugs	Smoke-free inhaled delivery systems for marijuana and cannabinoids
None recommended	Cigarettes and crude marijuana preparations should not be used	Novel cannabinoid analogs for new uses
None recommended	Not recommended	Smoke-free inhaled delivery system for marijuana and cannabinoids

[5]National Institutes of Health. 1997. Workshop on the medical utility of marijuana. Bethesda, MD: National Institutes of Health.

[6]British Medical Association. 1997. Therapeutic uses of cannabis. Harwood Academic Publishers, United Kingdom.

[7]Report of the Council on Scientific Affairs. 1997. Report to the AMA House of Delegates. Subject: Medical Marijuana.

symptoms and that more research on the medical use of marijuana is needed.

One recent report that does not appear in Table 12.1 is a 1996 publication from the Health Council of the Netherlands.[1] Unlike the six reports summarized in the table, the Health Council study concluded that not enough evidence existed to justify medical use of marijuana or THC, despite the fact that THC is an approved medicine in the United States (in the form of dronabinol) and in Britain (in the form of nabilone). It is important to note that the Health Council committee did not address the question of whether enough evidence exists to justify clinical trials of marijuana-based medicine. Instead, they were charged with determining whether marijuana or cannabinoids warrant prescription *in their current form*. And although they answered that question with a "no"—perhaps surprisingly since recreational use of marijuana has been decriminalized in the Netherlands—the Health Council noted that hospitals in the Netherlands tolerate marijuana use among patients with terminal illnesses. The council also said it "did not wish to judge patients who consume marihuana . . . because it makes them feel better."

While most of the reports in Table 12.1 spoke to the importance of developing smokeless delivery systems for cannabinoid medications, many echoed the IOM's conclusion that clinical trials of smoked marijuana may be appropriate until researchers develop safer ways to administer cannabinoids. Along with the IOM, the American Medical Association House of Delegates, the National Institutes of Health, and the British Medical Association have recommended clinical trials of smoked marijuana for much the same variety of symptoms.

The British Medical Association stated that marijuana itself is "unsuitable for medical practice" but nonetheless recommended that drug regulations be modified to facilitate research on the plant material. The British House of Lords report reached a similar conclusion, adding—in disagreement with the British Medical Association—that British doctors should be allowed to prescribe marijuana preparations until smokeless versions become available. Only the National Institutes of Health report recommends clinical studies of marijuana for the treatment of glaucoma.

In addition to considering reports from expert and governmental bodies, readers may be interested to learn what advocates both for and against the medical use of marijuana have to say on the subject. Every popular book with which we are familiar was written in support of the medical use of marijuana. For an opposing view, perhaps the best existing source is a scholarly review that appeared in the *Annals of Internal Medicine* in 1997.[2] Several major scientific and medical journals have reviewed the above publications, including most recently *Science*[3] and the *Journal of the American Medical Association*.[4]

INTO THE FUTURE

During the past two decades researchers have taken important steps toward understanding how cannabinoids exert their effects on the human body. These advances, summarized in Table 12.2, lay the foundation for the possible development of novel medicines from marijuana. Although the marijuana plant represents a rich source of cannabinoids, and of THC in particular, chemists are also synthesizing new versions of cannabinoids with properties that may improve their usefulness as medications, such as increased solubility in water.

In the early 1980s researchers had yet to determine whether THC acted on specific cellular receptors—as it is now known to do—or whether the cannabinoid acted nonspecifically, altering any cell with which it came in contact. The discovery of cannabinoid receptors means that it should be possible to design medicines that target the cells and tissues bearing the receptors. For example, researchers have found cannabinoid receptors in moderate abundance in areas of the brain and spinal cord that control pain perception and also in peripheral nerve cells, which detect pain sensations on the body 's surface. Perhaps a drug based on THC, which slows nerve impulses when it binds to one class of cannabinoid receptors, or a chemical derivative of that compound could be used to reduce pain sensations along these nerve pathways.

On the strength of these findings, along with the results of experiments in animals and a few clinical studies, the IOM study team concluded that cannabinoids hold particular promise as pain relievers. This is an instance where basic research has played

TABLE 12.2 Recent Discoveries in Cannabinoid Science

Year	Discovery
1986	Development of potent new synthetic cannabinoid compounds; they are the key to discovering the cannabinoid receptor.
1988	First conclusive evidence of specific receptors for cannabinoids.
1990	Cloning of a cannabinoid receptor from the brain (CB_1); this allows researchers to determine the sequence of the gene that encodes CB_1 and map the distribution of cannabinoid receptors throughout the brain.
1992	Discovery of anandamide, a naturally occurring substance in the brain that acts on cannabinoid receptors.
1993	Discovery of cannabinoid receptor outside the brain (CB_2) that is related to, but distinct from CB_1.
1994	Development of the first compound that specifically blocks cannabinoids from binding receptors.
1998	Development of a cannabinoid receptor blocker that binds CB_2 but not CB_1.

Source: Adapted from Institute of Medicine. 1999. *Marijuana and Medicine: Assessing the Science Base.* Washington, DC: National Academy Press, p. 34.

an especially important role in identifying potential new medicines. The opposite is true of evidence that cannabinoids can relieve nausea and vomiting, most of which comes from clinical studies of cancer patients undergoing chemotherapy. Scientists have a great deal to learn about the biological mechanisms that cause nausea and vomiting before they can attempt to identify ways to use cannabinoids to control these processes. And since highly effective antiemetic medicines already exist, there are far fewer incentives to develop cannabinoid drugs for nausea and vomiting than for other indications, such as pain.

In addition to pain, nausea, and vomiting, the IOM researchers identified appetite stimulation as a promising area for further development of marijuana-based medicines (i.e., in addition to oral THC). They also noted that some scientific evidence supports the possibility of treating muscle spasticity with cannabinoids but that these findings are neither especially strong nor consistent. For example, published reports fail to make the distinction between reducing muscle spasticity by inhibiting specific physiological processes or simply by relieving anxiety, which is known to exacerbate spastic symptoms. Even less evidence exists to indicate that cannabinoids might relieve movement disorders, the IOM report states, while noting encouraging results from relevant animal experiments.

Although researchers have yet to fully explore the variety of possible indications for marijuana-based medicines, one thing is clear: smoking marijuana is an inferior way to deliver its potential benefits. Marijuana smoke contains many of the same carcinogens and other harmful compounds found in tobacco smoke—agents that pose an even greater threat to people whose health is compromised by disease. Moreover, as is the case for other herbal remedies, whole marijuana plants contain variable mixtures of active compounds and are therefore likely to produce inconsistent results. Crude marijuana may also contain fungal spores and other potentially harmful contaminants that could pass into the respiratory tract. If there is any future in cannabinoid drugs, it lies in the safe, effective delivery of pure, active compounds.

To this end, several researchers and companies are pursuing the development of a smokeless inhaled delivery method for cannabinoid medications. For example, scientists at HortaPharm B.V.—a Dutch company that also grows research-grade marijuana for a variety of applications—are testing a device that gently heats marijuana, releasing a cannabinoid vapor that patients can inhale. A British firm, GW Pharmaceuticals Ltd., has licensed another technology, known as a nebulizer, that uses mechanical means to turn whole marijuana extracts into a fine mist. It is slated for use in upcoming individual trials to test the effectiveness of the extracts in patients with a variety of disorders, using a protocol similar to that recommended by the IOM for short-term trials of smoked marijuana.

Researchers have also submitted plans to Britain's Medical Research Council for two double-blind clinical trials to compare the effectiveness of inhaled marijuana extracts with oral THC and placebo. The first trial is expected to include 900 patients with multiple sclerosis who will test these treatments for their ability to relieve muscle spasticity. The second is a study of postoperative pain relief in 400 patients; it will also include a standard pain medication as a positive control. Both protocols were reviewed and approved, but at the time of writing only the multiple sclerosis trial had been funded.

Unfortunately, the very efficiency of cannabinoid inhalers raises the likelihood that they will be abused. Unlike oral THC, inhaled cannabinoids would probably rapidly produce the same "high" (or even a more powerful or potentially more addictive high) as smoking marijuana. Thus, manufacturers will probably need to build safeguards into cannabinoid inhalers to prevent their use for nonmedical purposes and also to limit the amount of drug the devices can deliver. These protective features can already be found in medical inhalers used to administer other controlled substances, including opiate painkillers.

Concern about possible abuse is but one of several barriers to developing medicines from marijuana or cannabinoids. As described in the previous two chapters, the issue of abuse has far-reaching economic and legal consequences, and the current status of marijuana as a Schedule I controlled substance represents a significant disincentive to both research and commercial development. Despite these odds, a few scientists and companies continue to pursue marijuana-based medicines. Since cannabinoid research is in its infancy, the possibility remains for future discoveries that inspire the development of important profitable drugs.

Rather than becoming blockbusters, however, it seems more likely that cannabinoid drugs will continue to be used in much the same way as oral THC: as alternatives or adjuncts to established therapies for a variety of symptoms. So far, conventional medicines have generally outperformed cannabinoid drugs in clinical trials. But not all medicines work for all people, so there may well be patients who will respond better to cannabinoids than to existing medications. And since cannabinoids appear to relieve some symptoms in novel ways, they could be combined with other drugs to enhance their effects. In particular, combinations of cannabinoids and opiates may prove to relieve pain better than opiates alone while causing fewer side effects.

It also appears that certain conditions may be uniquely suited to treatment with marijuana-based medicines. Most people with AIDS, for example, experience multiple symptoms that appear to be relieved by cannabinoids, including wasting, nausea, vomiting, pain, and anxiety. It might therefore be preferable to offer such patients a single medication that provides less-than-perfect relief for all of these symptoms than to treat each symptom with a different but more powerful drug.

Some of the most exciting possibilities that could unfold from our present medical knowledge of marijuana have little to do with the plant itself. The active compounds in marijuana may not only inspire scientists to develop a variety of useful synthetic medicines but also lead them to a greater understanding of the role of cannabinoids produced by the human body. Research has already revealed that cannabinoids influence numerous physiological processes and biochemical pathways, each of which represents a potential site of action for new highly specific drugs. With the advent of treatments designed to work with the body's own cannabinoid system, the medical use of marijuana should fade as a topic of heated debate to a footnote in the history of medicine.

NOTES

1. Health Council of the Netherlands, Standing Committee on Medicine. 1996. *Marihuana as Medicine.* Rijswikj, The Netherlands: Health Council of the Netherlands.

2. Voth EA, Schwartz RH. 1997. "Medicinal applications of delta-9-tetrahydrocannabinol and marijuana." *Annals of Internal Medicine* 126:791-798.

3. Hall W. 1997. "An ongoing debate." *Science* 278:75.

4. Strassman RJ. 1998. "Marihuana: The Forbidden Medicine" (book review). *Journal of the American Medical Association* 279:963-964.

INDEX

A

Addiction
  clinical studies, 47-48
  craving, 52, 53, 54
  epidemiological studies, 47-48,
    54, 57-58
  gateway theory, 5, 62-65, 67-68
  mental illness, 61
  tolerance, 11, 48, 49, 50, 52-53, 78
  withdrawal, 11, 41, 48, 49, 51-54
  see also Dependence
Adolescents, 51-52, 54, 65, 66
  attitudes, 66-67
  dependence, 56
  gateway theory, 63
  peer pressure, 54, 55, 63
Africa, 15
African Americans, 56
  glaucoma, 125
Age factors, 11
  AIDS, 86
  cellular biology of, 90
  clinical trials, 74
  elderly persons, 45, 74, 95, 125
  gateway theory, 63
  glaucoma, 124-125

prevalence of marijuana use, 54,
    56, 73
side effects of medication,
    general, 19-21
smoking of marijuana by
    patients, 90, 93, 161, 185
  see also Adolescents; Children
AIDS, 3, 4, 5, 7, 10, 19-20, 43, 44-45,
    86-94, 160, 164, 176-177,
    185
  age factors, 86
  clinical studies, 75, 84, 87-94, 134,
    135, 178-179
  Marinol, 88, 89-90, 91, 92, 134,
    135, 145
AIDS wasting, 8, 87-88, 101, 150,
    166, 185
  clinical studies, 84, 89-90, 93, 171
  Marinol, 27, 144, 145, 147
  patients' views, 19-21
  smoking of marijuana, 90, 93,
    161, 185
  THC, 108, 109, 111-113
Alaska, 4, 164
Alcohol use, 39, 56, 58, 60, 61
  gateway theory, 62-63, 64

C

D

04/16/2015